On Marijuana

Grafton and Scratch Publishers Canada
Grafton and Scratch Managment Inc.
onmarijuana@gmail.com

Printed in USA

Library and Archives Canada Cataloguing in Publication:

On marijuana : a powerful examination of what marijuana use means for our children, our communities, and our future / compiled by Pamela McColl.

Includes bibliographical references and index.
Issued in print and electronic formats.
ISBN 978-1-927979-07-5 (pbk.).—ISBN 978-1-927979-08-2 (epub).—ISBN 978-1-927979-09-9 (pdf)

1. Marijuana—Risk assessment. 2. Marijuana—Social aspects. 3. Marijuana—Health aspects. 4. Marijuana abuse. I. McColl, Pamela, 1958–, author, editor

HV5822.M3O55 2014 362.29′5 C2014-905910-8
C2014-905911-6

On Marijuana

A powerful examination of what marijuana use means for our children, our communities and our future

compiled by Pamela McColl
foreword by David Frum & Kevin A. Sabet, PhD

Contents

9 · Foreword

David Frum and Kevin A. Sabet, PhD

17 · Note to Reader

21 · Interview with Dr. David Musto from Frontline, "Busted: America's War on Marijuana"

Frontline/PBS Winter 1997-1998

49 · The Arguments for Legalization

Stuart Gitlow MD MPH MBA
President, American Society of Addiction Medicine

57 · What Canadian Youth Think About Cannabis: Report in Short

Canadian Centre on Substance Abuse (CCSA) September 2013
Amy J. Porath-Waller PHD, Jonathan E. Brown PHD,
Aarin P. Frigon MA, CHRP, Heath Clark MA

67 · What Are The Costs Associated with Marijuana Legalization?

Jo McGuire, Occupational Health & Safety September 2014

77 · The Pot Kids

David Berner, Executive Director, Drug Prevention Network of Canada, Therapist

89 · What Science Says About Marijuana

Samuel A. Ball, President and Chief Executive of CASA Columbia, University, and a professor of psychiatry at Yale Medical School.

91 · Statement Against Legalization of Marijuana

Hazelden Betty Ford Foundation

95 · Drug Free Australia's Position on Medical Marijuana/Cannabis

July 2014

109 · Legalization Always Increases Use

Edward Gogek MD

115 · What is the Societal Impact of Legalized Marijuana?

Lynette Crow-Iverson, Conspire!

129 · An Example of Marijuana's Impact on Teen Brain Activity

Dr. Andra Smith PHD Associate Professor, School of Psychology, University of Ottawa, Canada

141 · Mixing Cannabis and Alcohol

National Cannabis Prevention and Information Centre

145 · An Open Letter to States Considering Legalization of Marijuana

Ed Wood, President, DUID Victim Voices

149 · Cannabis: General Facts An Extract from Cannabis: A General Survey of its Harmful Effects

Updated 2014:10

Mary Brett, Chair CanSS, member of the World Forum Against Drugs

173 · How Physicians Should Respond to the New Cannabis Regulations

Canadian Journal of Addiction 2013:9

Meldon Kahan MD CCFP and Sheryl Spithoff MD CCFP

197 · Marijuana and Pregnancy: What Are the Risks?

Pamela McColl, Director and Advisory Council Member to Smart Approaches to Marijuana Canada

203 · Cannabis and the Reproductive System, Pregnancy and the Development of Children

Mary Brett, Chair CanSS, member of the World Forum Against Drugs

235 · Silent Forests? Rodenticides on Illegal Marijuana Crops Harm Wildlife

Wildlife Society News Spring 2013

Mourad W. Gabriel, Greta M. Wengert, J.Mark Higley, Shane Krogan, Warren Sargent, Deana L. Clifford

249 · Changes in Attitudes, Intentions, and Behaviors toward Tobacco and Marijuana during US Students' First Year of College Tobacco Use Insights.
Mara W. Stewart, Megan A. Moreno MD, MPH,MSED

279 · Marijuana: Medicine, Addictive Substance, or Both? A Common-Sense Approach to the Place of Cannabis in Medicine
Canadian Journal of Addiction 2013:9
Harold Kalant CM, MD, PhD, FRSC Professor Emeritus, University of Toronto

293 · Finding Solutions
Robert B. Charles, former Assistant Secretary of State, for International Narcotics and Law Enforcement Affairs (INL)

305 · The Nature and Extent of Marijuana Possession in British Columbia
Kale Pauls RCMP, Dr. Irwin M. Cohen, Dr. Darryl Plecas, Tara Haarhoff, RCMP

Foreword

Marijuana. Cannabis. Pot. Nowadays these terms often preclude some tense argument or shouting match pertaining to health and safety, therapeutic value, societal responses, and legalization policy. Popular websites and blogs, user forums, television news specials, Facebook postings and tweets are filled with information about how marijuana is a relatively benign herb, having endured a century of suffering at the hands of evil government doers.

But what is rarely said or spoken about, it seems, is what scientists and historians have to say about the drug. It is not often that the positions of the Canadian or American Medical Associations, the World Health Organization, or the evidence gathered and published in prestigious works like the New England Journal of Medicine are broadcast widely, let alone translated into words most people can easily grasp. Half-second Google searches will show plenty of results about how marijuana is harmless; it takes a deep dive, however, to grasp the 0.01 p-level significance of large longitudinal studies examining the complex interaction between IQ and heavy marijuana use, for example.

Add to this a relentless campaign by would-be profiteers to commercialize and legitimize marijuana and you get the situation society seems to be in now: a tangled confusion about marijuana's true health harms, the risks to society if use spreads, and the potential of a for-profit commercial market to advertise and promote heavy abuse.

This book helps to rid the debate of that confusion. It presents, plainly and openly, the harms numerous reputable researchers and organizations are concerned about. This is required reading for officials contemplating marijuana legalization.

It is also remarkable that now we have some concrete examples of legalization—no longer is legalization just a theory or idea. It has now been implemented in a handful of jurisdictions in North America.

After multimillion-dollar political campaigns, Colorado and Washington voters legalized marijuana in November of 2012. Though it would take more than a year to set up retail stores, personal use (in Colorado and Washington) and home cultivation and giving away of up to 6 plants (in Colorado) were almost immediately legalized following the vote. Public marijuana use, though illegal, remains a common way to celebrate the law, and a brand new industry selling candies, waxes, sodas, and other marijuana items exploded.

The US federal government announced they would initially take a hands-off approach, promising to track nine consequences (from youth marijuana use to use on public lands) and determine action later. So far, however, no robust public tracking system by federal or state authorities has been implemented. The group Smart Approaches to Marijuana (SAM), one that we helped to establish in 2013, began tracking developments on a website www.legalizationviolations.com, along with its main home, www.learnaboutsam.org.

And though it is too early to firm up final conclusions, there are concerns in 2015 we cannot ignore after two full years of legalized possession and one year of legalized retail sales.

- Past-year and past-month marijuana use by all ages exceeds the national average in both Washington State and Colorado. Marijuana use in both these states has risen significantly between 2011-2012 and 2012-2013.
- Between 2008 and 2011, an average of 4 children (between the ages of 3 and 7) were sent to the ER for unintentional marijuana ingestion. In 2013, 8 children went to the Colorado Children's hospital. As of the first half of 2014, at least 14 children have already been sent to the ER.
- According to the Washington Poison Center, "the selling of cannabis for recreational purposes became legalized in the state of Washington on July 7th, 2014. As a direct result, the Washington Poison Center (WAPC) has encountered an increase in the number of human exposures related to accidental or excessive consumption/

...halation of marijuana and marijuana edibles, particularly among pediatrics."

- Edibles often contain more than three to twenty times the THC concentration recommended for intoxication. Manufacturing practices are not yet standardized in CO or WA, and childproof packaging remains a challenge. There have been at least 2 deaths related to marijuana edibles in 2014, and state officials still cannot agree on how to regulate them.
- Contaminant testing in Washington finds that 13% of pot and THC-infused products contain mold, salmonella, and E. coli. Colorado has not begun such testing yet.
- A marijuana-focused private equity firm, Privateer Holdings in partnership with the descendants of Bob Marley, have created a multinational cannabis brand called Marley Natural. Investors have already raised $50 million to launch Marley Natural.

Interestingly, however, these statistics might be prompting the beginning of a backlash. Hidden beneath the headlines of the American elections in 2014 was the fact that 26 out of 31 localities in Colorado voted to prohibit marijuana stores outright. Many of these localities had voted for the legalization ballot measure two years prior. And a Gallup poll taken in October of 2014 showed a 7 percentage point drop in the number of Americans supporting legalization – from 58% to 51%. Surely, legalization advocates – fueled now by a growing, profitable industry – are going to double down and move full steam ahead with their plans to legalize drugs.

As we are beginning to see, the promise that legalization will actually protect teenagers from marijuana is false. So, too, are the other promises of the legalizers. It is false to claim that marijuana legalization will break drug cartels. Those cartels will continue to traffic in harder and more lucrative drugs, such as heroin, cocaine, and methamphetamine. Criminal cartels may well stay in the marijuana business, too, marketing directly to underage users. In fact, the black market has thrived in Colorado.

Public policy is about trade-offs, and marijuana users need to face up to the trade-off they are urging on North American society. Legal marijuana use means more marijuana use, and more marijuana use means above all more teen marijuana use.

Some older adults have a hard time crediting the dangers of marijuana use because they imagine the marijuana on sale today is the same low-grade stuff they smoked in college. The marijuana sold in the 1980s averaged between 3 and 4 percent THC, the psychoactive ingredient. Today's selectively bred marijuana averages over 12 percent THC, with some strains reaching 30 percent. Hundreds of YouTube videos will show you how to combust a marijuana wax with butane, to boost the THC content to 90 percent. As marijuana consumers shift from smoking to ingesting marijuana, they can ingest larger and larger doses of THC at a time. Since 2006, Colorado emergency rooms have seen a steep rise in the number of patients arriving panicked and disoriented from excess THC, including a near doubling of patients ages 13 and 14. It's said that nobody ever died from a marijuana overdose. Nobody ever died from a tobacco overdose either, but that doesn't prove tobacco safe.

Lucrative industries have arisen to exploit these weaknesses in ways highly harmful to their customers. And the bold irony is that when their practices are challenged, they'll invoke the very principles of individual choice and self-mastery that their industry is based on negating and defeating. So it was with tobacco. So it is with casino gambling. So it will be with marijuana.

Proponents of marijuana legalization do make a valid point when they worry that marijuana laws are enforced too punitively—and that this too punitive approach inflicts disparate punishment on minority users as compared with white users. Ordinary marijuana users should receive civil penalties; repeat users belong in treatment, not prison; communities should experience law enforcement as an ally and supporter of local norms, not an outside force stamping people with indelible criminal records for mistakes that carry fewer consequences for the more affluent and the better connected. It's also true, however, that these alternative methods can succeed only if the background rule is that marijuana is illegal. It's very often the threat of criminal sanction that impels users to seek the treatment they need, while still young enough to turn their lives around.

If marijuana is legalized, what will emerge is an industry that serves the market will be emboldened to hire lobbyists to promote its continued expansion. The vision offered by some academics of a legal but noncommercial marijuana market shows little realism about American government. American legislatures exhibit notoriously poor resistance against checkbook-wielding special interests.

The resistance will be all the weaker since the costs of marijuana legalization will be borne by people to whom political leadership pay scant attention anyway. Marijuana retailers will be located most densely in our poorest neighborhoods, just as liquor and cigarette retailing is now. Out of whose pockets will the marijuana taxes of the future be paid? Whose addiction and recovery services will be least well funded? In a society in which it is already sufficiently difficult for people to rise from the bottom, who'll find that their rise has become harder still?

These are tough questions that deserve contemplation, not bumper sticker slogans. Voters and decision makers alike would do well to at least educate themselves first on the potential ramifications of a "pot-for-all" policy. This book will help them do that.

David Frum and Kevin A. Sabet, PhD

Note to Reader

MARIJUANA USE HAS adverse consequences on the health, well-being, and safety of both individual users and nonusers. The evidence is clear that marijuana use places a heavy burden on social systems, taxes the economy, and places a heavy strain on public health care resources.

On Marijuana is a powerful examination of what marijuana use really means for our children, our communities, and our future. It contains insightful, considered opinions from individuals who have dedicated themselves, and often their lengthy careers, to the study and better understanding of the implications, risks, and effects of using marijuana products. *On Marijuana* is a not for profit publication. Any profits generated from sales of *On Marijuana* will be employed to distribute this publication to the public sector. The soft cover and eBook publications of On Marijuana are available on internet book retail sites worldwide. For further information contact the publisher at onmarijuana@gmail.com

Many thanks to: Gerilee McBride and Ron Kirkish and to all the authors who either gave reprint rights or wrote especially for this publication. Thank you also goes to other publications and publishers who graciously granted reprint rights.

Disclaimer

The information provided in this book is designed to provide helpful information on the subjects discussed. This book is not meant to be used, nor should it be used, to diagnose or treat any medical condition. For diagnosis or treatment of any medical problem, consult your own physician. References are provided for informational purposes only and do not constitute endorsement of any websites or other sources.

It is sold or given with the understanding that the publisher is not engaged to render any type of psychological, legal, or any other kind of professional advice. The content of each article is the sole expression and opinion of its authors, and not necessarily that of the publisher. No warranties or guarantees are expressed or implied by the publisher's choice to include any of the content in this volume. Neither the publisher nor the individual author(s) shall be liable for any physical, psychological, emotional, financial, or commercial damages, including, but not limited to, special, incidental, consequential or other damages.

While best efforts have been used in preparing this book, the authors and publisher make no representations or warranties of any kind and assume no liabilities of any kind with respect to the accuracy or completeness of the contents. Neither the author nor the publisher shall be held liable or responsible to any person or entity with respect to any loss or incidental or consequential damages caused, or alleged to have been caused, directly or indirectly, by the information herein.

Further articles and contact details are available on the books' website *www.onmarijuana.info*

The Publisher

DR. DAVID F. MUSTO
Yale University
(1936–2010)

Interview with Dr. David Musto from *Frontline*, "Busted: America's War on Marijuana" (Winter 1997–1998)

Interviewer

Can you outline marijuana's history in the U.S.?

Dr. David Musto

Marijuana started to come into the United States in the 1920s along with Mexican immigrants, who worked in the beet fields, in the gardens, and so on. Some of the first anti-marijuana laws, occurred in, somewhat unusual places, such as Arizona, Colorado, Idaho, Michigan. And this is because the Mexican immigrants did grow marijuana and did use marijuana and it caused some concern among the people in the vicinity.

Then in the 1930s, when the Great Depression hit, these people became a feared surplus in our country. People tried to get them to go back to Mexico. They were thought to be undercutting Americans for jobs, and they were thought to take marijuana, go into town on the weekends, for example, and create mayhem. Now that's very close to the general attitude toward marijuana in the 1930s … that marijuana released inhibitions, and caused people to act, and, to perhaps, be violent. Even researchers, who were most calm, so to speak, about marijuana saw it as a very serious problem with regard to releasing inhibitions.

Interviewer
Was this based on real evidence, or was it coming out of a personal attitude toward the people?

Dr. David Musto
It's hard to say. It is what researchers saw when they looked at marijuana. And I know one researcher, who lived in the 1930s, and has lived until today, and he, himself, [says] what a strange thing it was. Because he now sees marijuana so differently, something that leads certainly not to a release of inhibitions, and a sort of violent way. And he puzzles himself, as to why was it looked at one way at one time, and now it's looked at a different way. So I can't quite explain it, except it was thought to be a cause of crime and a cause of senseless violence in the 1930s.

Now, how to control something that was in fact a weed, something that had been grown in the United States for hemp since the 18th century was a real problem. And the head of the narcotics bureau, Harry J. Anslinger, really did not want, in his heart, a federal anti- marijuana law. Because he saw it as putting a tremendous burden on the Federal Bureau of Narcotics [FBN]. They got no more money, they got no more agents, and they're supposed to stamp out a weed. He was telling me that once he was driving across a bridge in the upper Potomac, he stopped his car, and he got out, and he says, there it was—marijuana, as far as you could see it on this river. And he said, "This, they want me to stamp out."

What Anslinger wanted was a uniform state narcotics law, so that each state would enact a law, presumably against marijuana. Now Anslinger was not for marijuana, but each state would decide, for itself, how much resources it wanted to spend in fighting marijuana. He worked with this, but it didn't happen. And then there's quite a bit of pressure on the Treasury Department and the administration to come up with something about marijuana because there was a growing pressure for anti-marijuana legislation from the west and from the southwest.

Then a curious thing happened. The National Firearms Act, was upheld by the Supreme Court, I think, it was February, 1937. The National Firearms Act was very strange because it attacked machine guns by saying you could not give somebody a machine gun, or loan them a machine gun, until you had first purchased a machine gun transfer stamp. And the government did not make any machine gun transfer stamps. So this was their way of trying to control machine guns.

Well, it was upheld by the Supreme Court, and within a month later, the treasury was in to Congress saying they wanted a marijuana tax stamp act, in which you could not give, barter, sell, or whatever it is marijuana unless first, you got a marijuana tax stamp. And an ordinary person could not get a marijuana tax stamp. So, that is how we got the initial marijuana law in 1937, and it was actually over the best judgment of the head of the bureau of narcotics, who really wanted to just deal with heroin, and cocaine, and opium, things that came from abroad. He did not want to deal with things that were indigenous to the United States.

Interviewer
Why did he do that?

Dr. David Musto
He had experience as assistant commissioner of Prohibition up until about 1930, that when you dealt with a domestic problem, you might arrest a local druggist, or the local doctor, [and] you got into a lot of difficulty. Also, you had problems with the federal courts. The federal courts would say, "Why are you in here with the minor case of someone dealing with alcohol?" It would be embarrassing and the judges would be difficult with them. And he thought the success of his bureau would depend upon being careful about what you were controlling. He did not want to control things that involved him with domestic issues in this way. He preferred to deal with something that came from abroad, and when you caught somebody with it you had done something that everyone was proud of.

Now, of course, they still went after doctors and pharmacists, with regard to cocaine, heroin, or opium, ... but the American people were so fearful of these substances that there was really very little complaint when someone was put out of business for a giving out cocaine, something like that. And, in fact, Anslinger worked very hard to prevent the FBN from ever having [to deal with] amphetamines, or barbiturates, or these other kinds of substances which are now controlled. He wanted a very lean, simple, administration.

There's one other point I might make, and that is, he had a very small budget, the budget was only $2 million a year or so, and he would be cross-examined by Congress when he spoke before them as to how much he had spent on long distance telephone calls, for example. It was a very difficult time—the Depression. And so he was more than impressed with the difficulties he would have trying to control marijuana without any more money, without any more agents.

So what Anslinger decided he had to do is fight marijuana in the media. And so he tried to describe marijuana in so repulsive and terrible terms that people wouldn't even be tempted to try it. He did something else that was quite interesting. There were people going around the country alarming parents about the use of marijuana among their children. These people he tried to shut down.

It's quite interesting because once the law was passed, if there were any great agitation about marijuana, in the country, there was only one person to come to and complain to, and that would be Anslinger, and there was not much he could do about it. So actually, what he wanted, was silence on marijuana, but if you had to know something about it, what you would learn is that it was a most terrible, violent, repulsive thing, and you wouldn't want to try it once.

So he fought his battle against marijuana in the media, you might say, because it was the cheapest thing he could possibly do, and he had no money to do anything else with.

Interviewer
Give me some examples. How did he portray it and in what way?

Dr. David Musto
Marijuana was portrayed as a substance that if you used marijuana, you might suddenly run amok, you might stab and kill people. They really described, what you might call the paranoia of cocaine psychosis, but they attributed it to smoking marijuana. And that if you did smoke marijuana, there was an extremely dangerous situation and you might, on the street, just simply see somebody and think they were after you and kill them.

There was a time in the hearings in which they had a color photograph of somebody who was beaten to death by someone who was said to be on marijuana. And they showed this to the committee. The committee misunderstood it, they thought, "This is what you look like if you took marijuana." And it had to be explained to them, "No, this is what someone on marijuana did to someone else under the haze of this drug." So, violence and release of inhibitions was the theme of marijuana in the 1930s.

And, I've always thought that it reveals how much the general attitude we have toward a substance affects [and] the research that is done on it. Because in the 1930s, almost no research could be found which in any way would reassure you about marijuana. But in the 1960s, when I was at the National Institute of Mental Health, there was almost no research that was done that could find anything wrong with marijuana.

So you have these enormous shifts and research, [that] takes place against these larger attitudes and it's also interpreted in these larger attitudes. So marijuana is an excellent example of how we have shifted our views on a substance.

[The] image of marijuana [created by the government in the 1930s eventually] did [the] government great damage in the 1960s. Because when people started using marijuana and they did not become insane to any great degree, that completely undercut the government's image of drugs. And there were people in the 60s, early 70s, who if the government warned them about something, like say, methamphetamine or speed, they would think, "This must be a good thing to try." The government had really lost its credibility ... what Anslinger did and what other people did in the 30s was all, they thought, for the sake of the people and of the public and so on, but it really, in the long run, backfired against the government.

Interviewer

What specific means did Anslinger use in the media?

Dr. David Musto

The newspapers and magazines were his primary outlet for information on marijuana ... [there] was a very interesting story on the movies. Anslinger was delighted, in 1934, when the Motion Pictures Association of America, made it forbidden to show any narcotics in films. That had been a very great criticism of films in the 1920s, that narcotics use was shown and even how to use narcotics.

So, in 1934 the Major Motion Pictures Studios established a production code, and you couldn't get a seal of approval if there were any narcotics in the motion picture. So actually you couldn't use films.

And eventually this upset him very much, because the Federal Bureau of Investigation, which was his model of how he wanted the FBN to be, was getting all kinds of good publicity, and people like, Jimmy Cagney and Humphrey Bogart, were becoming FBI agents in the movies. And there couldn't be any narcotics agents in the movies because he had succeeded in getting narcotics taken out of the movies.

Finally, in 1948, he got slight modification that you could show the narcotics agents and a motion picture was made, called "To The Ends of The Earth" with Dick Powell. And that does show the narcotics bureau. But no films were really out for him. And that was because they wanted the public to know nothing about narcotics, you see? Silence, was a very important element of the drug strategy, in the 1930s and 40s and 50s. The drug problem had been greater, it had gone way down, and they didn't want to wake sleeping dogs, so to speak.

And, when it did start to come up again, when heroin started to be used again in the 50s, in New York and in Chicago and among younger people, and in Hispanic and in black neighborhoods, the thing they reached for was increased penalties. Anslinger had tremendous faith in penalties as a way of controlling things.

In the 1950s, when there was a concern about heroin, the laws were strengthened and they introduced mandatory sentences, and they included marijuana in these mandatory minimum sentences. It was thought that if you had very severe laws on the books, it would discourage the pubic from trying these drugs, or using them to any great extent.

Now there's a curious story about that, because in the first drug epidemic which peaked around, World War I, say 1900-1915, we had no laws against drugs until the public demanded laws against drugs. And when the public demanded laws against drugs, it meant we had a consensus in the country against drugs. People were very frightened by them. They [drugs] had been very easily available, we were the only country really to have a free economy in drugs in the 19th century. But that caused quite a bit of concern about drugs, and the effects of all this drug use. So when the laws came into effect during the first epidemic, they seemed to be very powerful, because they came right along with the decline in drug use.

But in the second epidemic, the one we're in now, we had the most severe drug laws on the books that you could have! Including the death penalty after 1956. And we still have a drug epidemic. So, our current view of laws and drugs is a little bit different than it was for people of Anslinger's time, who really thought that the whole story was the laws. Because, actually, I think it's much more reasonable to say that the laws could help to some extent, and they had some value. But the real change of attitude was the attitude among the public which became very anti-drug and very fearful of drugs.

Interviewer
What was creating the public attitude, though?

Dr. David Musto
We have in this country a pattern of looking at drugs and other substances, such as food, almost as an instrument to improve ourselves. To give an example of this—during each of the great anti-drug or temperance movements in this country, there's also been a very strong health movement at the same time. So these big movements that we talk about actually relate to what we think of the environment, and what we take into our bodies.

And we became very concerned about what we take into our bodies during what you might call a temperance period or an anti-drug period. And that goes back each time we've had one of these in our history. So what we call an anti-drug movement, you could, at the same time, call it a pro-health movement in which people become very concerned. One example—Jerry Rubin, somebody I got to know in the 60s. He was familiar with, I think, all drugs known to mankind. And in the 60s, people looked upon drugs as instruments that would help them achieve something that they couldn't achieve by themselves. They were an aid in some way. Then after about 1980, the attitude started to shift. And people started to think that if you take drugs, you're reduced by that much. Jerry Rubin moved from trying any drug that was around, to having a dietitian come to his house, twice a week, to plan out the most healthy possible food there could be.

In other words, he made the perfect transition from the 60s, which was tolerant of anything, to the 1980s and 90s in which there's a great concern about what we take into our body and are we healthy and are we exercising properly and so on. So, in a way, these large movements have to do with our attitude toward risk. And we move from risk-taking, to risk-reduction. And many things follow in that, including drugs, health, foods we eat, and so on.

Interviewer
Do you think of marijuana as particularly symbolic regarding American ambivalence about drugs?

Dr. David Musto
Well, marijuana in the 30s was symbolic of Mexican immigrants, let's say, who were feared and were seen as a uneconomic surplus. And in the 1960s, when people took marijuana, it was seen as a symbol of belonging to something which was very moral, and was fighting the establishment. So you see that marijuana in both instances, as drugs often do, symbolized something larger.

You can either take a drug, because it symbolizes something, or you can refuse to take a drug that symbolizes something. When I first started work on this many years ago, the first big surprise I got was the way in which cocaine became symbolic of southern blacks and the period before World War I. And the tremendous fear of blacks and cocaine. I had never heard of this before. Then in the 30s we have marijuana and Mexican immigrants. We also had smoking opium and Chinese immigrants. So you often have a drug that is symbolically linked to some feared group.

It could go the other way, too. I remember that when Ghandi, in his experiments on truth, wrote about [how] he was trying to figure out why the British were so tall and so strong. And he decided [it was] because they eat meat. And although he very later became a very strict vegetarian, he did try to eat meat. And so substances can symbolize, positively or negatively. And marijuana has symbolized both. To some people, it has symbolized the best in the opportunities we have in the future—to change people and to make them more cooperative and empathetic. And to other people, marijuana has come to symbolize the decay of society and, perhaps, violence and danger.

Interviewer
Almost like two sides of America ...

Dr. David Musto
That's right. American has both of these images. America has

both the image of being very strict, [for example], national prohibition. Very few countries ever had national prohibition. We had it for almost 14 years. And on the other hand, we're a country that's famous for heavy drinking at various times around the time of the 18th, 19th century, and about 1830, we drank, per capita, three to four times what we drink per capita now in alcohol. So the United States has both of these images—has the image of prohibition and abstinence, and it has the image of tolerance of drugs and whatever you want to take and as much as you want to take.

Interviewer
Where are we right now?

Dr. David Musto
When you go to graduate school for history, you have to take an oath against predicting the future. I don't want to be thrown out of the American Historical Association, but I would say that the peak of our toleration of drugs was reached about 1979 or 1980.

And since then, in general, we have been becoming more and more anti-drug. We've become more anti-alcohol. Alcohol consumption hit a peak in 1980 also, as well as marijuana hit a peak, about 1980. So, in many ways, we're becoming more strict. If you look at the laws on the books that have been passed, in 1986 and 1988, the Anti-Drug Abuse Acts, the fact that we now have warning labels on alcohol beverage containers and the drinking age raised to 21. Various things happening. The great acceptance of drug testing, for example. All of these things are increasingly accepted, because we are more in agreement against drugs such as marijuana.

Now that is a particular complexity for marijuana because marijuana is used by a great many people. And I think that, actually, the American people are, in a way, deciding now about marijuana in a way that they could have never had the opportunity before. We are, in a sense, in the process of mulling over what we are going to do about marijuana, but when we looked at our attitude toward tobacco, and how that has accelerated, and how we're really moving toward the prohibition of tobacco. It may not happen, but we're pretty close to it now. And then you compare that attitude with what we should do about marijuana. You can see that this is in a period of much greater concern, and the desire to control, then let's say the 1960s.

Interviewer
What about the medical marijuana debate?

Dr. David Musto
The medical marijuana debate is extremely interesting. There's no question that people who want to legalize marijuana are using the medical marijuana issue as a wedge, and something like that had been tried earlier with heroin, for the terminally ill. That is the idea being, if you can get one of these feared drugs to be seen as a medicine, then it's not that far to saying well, perhaps we should regulate its use rather than prohibit its use.

On the other hand, there are many statements from people who have used marijuana in situation in which they've been greatly helped by marijuana and that's in their testimony. So it's quite difficult. You have, on the one hand, the actual medical benefits of marijuana, which are debated and then you have it being used as a wedge. I think that it would be quite possible to do studies that would confirm, so to speak, once and for all, what is the value of marijuana as an anti-nausea medication or as an anti-glaucoma medication. I've been told by an opthamologist that if you wanted to take marijuana for glaucoma, you have to smoke five or six joints a day every day of your life. Well, if that's true, and I don't know if that's true, that's a very different way of saying it's useful in glaucoma, then people usually take one drop, in their eye of another medication.

So I think that medical marijuana is quite an interesting issue, and it brings up one other point I would like to make. And that is, before basic narcotics law in this country, which was the Harrision Act in 1915, all the states had different drug policies. For example, Massachusetts did not allow heroin maintenance; New York state set up clinics to provide morphine maintenance. That's how enormously different the states were.

Well, we may be unraveling the national consensus on drugs, and bringing back to the states the decision as to what to do with drugs. Because the votes in Arizona and in California, suggest that their could be part of the country in which there's a different point of view. And I don't know exactly how that would take place, but for someone from a historical point of view, it's extremely interesting because the Harrision Act was considered a great achievement because it harmonized all of these state laws. But now, we may be going back to the situation where each state will decide for itself what it wants to do about some substances like marijuana, which is what Anslinger wanted to have happen in the first place!

Interviewer
Returning to some history again—marijuana was associated with jazz, black jazz music.

Dr. David Musto
That's true. There's some evidence that jazz bands actually spread the use of marijuana and were a source of marijuana in the town that they went to. Now this is an allegation that's been made. I've never checked this out, but Anslinger said to me once "We had more jazz bands in jail in the 1930s than I can count." Now I didn't know whether this was just hyperbole and there's no way really to check these things, but there were well-known band leaders who wrote music for marijuana, including Benny Goodman and others, songs were recorded, were available, and this was another bane of Anslinger, the idea that marijuana made you play jazz better.

And there was even a study done, in which they recorded people playing jazz under marijuana, playing jazz without marijuana, and the jazz played without marijuana was much better than the jazz played with marijuana. This is the kind of scientific studies that were being done. And jazz bands— we'll take, Louie Armstrong, who is said to have never stopped using marijuana in his lifetime.

In general, the whole attitude toward the substance became more negative. So, for example, in '46 or '47, Robert Mitchum was arrested for marijuana use and had to spend 30 days in the Los Angeles prison farm doing something. There was no talk about it at that time, about [how] he shouldn't have to do this or this was excessive, or anything like this. It was actually shocking news. That this had happened to most of the public. So whereas marijuana might have been seen as bohmeian kind of use of the drug in the 20s and the 30s, it gradually became something that was practically equated with heroin or cocaine.

Interviewer
World War II—was there a big shift in the government's attitude towards marijuana?

Dr. David Musto
Well, what happened during World War II was that we were cut off from our supply of rope and the Navy needed ropes. And we had grown hemp in this country in the 18th century; John Adams promoted it very strongly from Massachusetts and said this would be a great new American economic crop. So the Federal Bureau of Narcotics gave licenses to a number of farmers to grow hemp to make rope. It turned out the rope was not very good, it isn't easy to make good rope and it

failed. Anslinger told me that he gave out these licenses to farmers in the northern areas, like Minnesota, because he felt they wouldn't know what they were planting, and he wanted to avoid giving it to people like in Kentucky who knew exactly what they would be planting. I'm not sure this is exactly correct because I think there was some marijuana or hemp being grown for the fiber in Kentucky at that time, but the government didn't reverse its attitude toward marijuana. But what it needed was the hemp fibers for the Navy.

Interviewer
Speaking of hemp, I've heard what partly motivated the original laws against marijuana was William Randolph Hearst, who wanted to have a monopoly on paper manufacturing. Hemp was in competition for paper.

Dr. David Musto
There have been some unusual explanations of why we had the Marijuana Tax Act. The first one I remember having heard in the 60s was the alcohol industry just got through prohibition, and they realized that if you could grow marijuana in your backyard,[it] would cost you simply nothing to get high, you wouldn't buy alcohol. So the alcohol industry was behind the Marijuana Tax Act.

Then I've heard, it was actually the DuPont Company, because the DuPont Company was coming out with nylon, and they were very fearful of competition from hemp, which was also very strong fiber. Therefore, the DuPont Company was behind the Marijuana Tax Act. And then there's the argument that William Randolph Hearst was really behind the Act because he had paper plantations and trees to make paper and you could also make paper out of hemp and therefore he wanted to get rid of hemp.

And I've looked into these; there's no evidence that they were correct. I think they come from people who can't believe that you could actually just be against marijuana just because it's marijuana.

And the Marijuana Tax Act, which I've looked into at great length, is fully explained by this agitation, which really was linked to the fear of Mexican immigrants and the pressures on the government, and then they're using the National Firearms Act model to form the Marijuana Tax Act. And I see no evidence that either William Randolph Hearst, the DuPont Company, or the liquor industry was behind it. But I would say about every five or six years a new explanation comes up.

Interviewer

In a way, this whole debate over marijuana continually seems to bring in all these other themes in American politics. It seems pretty much like a trigger point.

Dr. David Musto

Yes, it had become that. When marijuana was outlawed, the congressmen who were in these committees and so on, really didn't know anything about it. They were very unfamiliar with it and they were taking the government's word for it.

And I think, subsequently, it has become a different kind of a problem because now you have a sizable number of people who say marijuana is OK and then you have an often other sizable number of people who say it isn't OK.

You really do get into all sorts of areas as to how we should lead our lives. Much of the debate over drugs comes from the philosophy of life. How should you live your life? Should you lead it in a rather controlled, disciplined way? Productive? Thinking about the future? So on and so forth? Or should you think about just today and the important thing is relationships with people rather than thinking ahead. Should the government intrude on your private right to do something? Or does the government have an obligation to take steps to protect you in ways that you couldn't protect yourself?

This goes back to the federalist papers, or to the Constitution ... and marijuana has become the symbol of how we should think about something, whether it's a medicine or not a medicine, a private right or a public right. And it is very rich—the whole discussion on marijuana is fascinating because people bring to it their deepest feelings and their image of how they would like the world to be run.

Both world views are American. If you want to look back into American history, you can find both sides well represented at various times in our history, and how this is going to work out it's hard to predict. But I would say that the fight over tobacco ... [there] must be a lot there to learn with regard to marijuana.

How people have come to see tobacco and secondary

smoke and so on the great alarm over this you wonder how much would be transferred to the issue of marijuana. At the moment, they really seem to be considered separate, but it's hard to imagine they can stay separate indefinitely.

Interviewer

What was happening in terms of research into marijuana at the end of the 60s?

Dr. David Musto

Well, there was a lot of interest in doing research on marijuana in the late 60s as the Nixon administration was very interested in doing something about drugs and trying to get the NIMH to do more research in this. And out of the 1970 Comprehensive Drug Abuse Act, came a request that there be established a commission to look into marijuana and drug abuse in general.

That was called the Shafer Commission because Governor Shafer of Pennsylvania chaired it. Well, they came out with the conclusion that marijuana should be decriminalized, that small amounts for personal use might be fined like you might get a ticket. People who were involved in big transportation of it would still be arrested and go to jail. And this was very upsetting to President Nixon.

Now, President Nixon, I think of all of our presidents, was the one most viscerally opposed to drugs. And he was very upset at the result of the Shafer Commission and I remember he refused to allow any pictures to be taken or be seen receiving this first report of the Shafer Commission, which was bound in a green covered document entitled "Marijuana: Symbol Of Misunderstanding," if I recall correctly. And the Shafer Commission was quite interesting because it started off with people who seemed quite conservative on the marijuana issue and wound up with this position, which is still considered a rather liberal position.

So, Nixon did not accept this and what he did was set up large amounts of treatment and research and other things for drugs. And the decriminalization idea in the Shafer Commission didn't arise again until the Carter administration. And [during] the Carter administration, I think it was in 1978, all the heads of the agencies came before Congress and asked for the decriminalization of marijuana of up to one ounce and it was quite interesting. There was quite a backlash to this.

The National Organization for the Reform of Marijuana Laws had been formed in 1970. They were very upset about what experts were saying about marijuana, they were very upset about people having enormously long minimum sentences for the possession of marijuana and they got quite agitated over it. At the end of the 70s, you had the parents movement formed and by this time drug experts were saying marijuana is just a stage of life, it's nothing to be excited about and so on. And the parents movement got very excited at the new batch of experts and they created quite a reaction and defeated some people who were running for Congress and had favored decriminalization. And then President Carter's drug advisor had to resign after having written a prescription with a false name on it. And so the Carter administration represents both the peak of decriminalization of marijuana and attempts to do it and also the beginning of the decline in support for marijuana.

And so you move right from the Carter administration into the Reagan administration, which was very anti-drug and anti-marijuana. So, the decriminalization things came out first I think in `72 with the first report of marijuana commission, reached a peak about 1978 or so and has been in decline, pretty much, since then.

Interviewer
Were parents a major force in the creation of the 1986 law?

Dr. David Musto
Yes. The parents movement became very strong, they were perceived as very strong by the Carter administration, the last two years of the Carter administration and during all of the Reagan administration. In fact, the parents movement got into a position where they were able to review the publications of the National Institute on Drug Abuse and were able to stop publications which waffled on attitudes towards drugs. They wanted a very clear no-tolerance position presented in any government publication, as well as any place else.

And so the parents' movement was perceived by politicians as an important representative group of Americans who demanded more action ... about 1986 and the crack epidemic and the death of Len Bias and all that sort of thing lead to this tremendous desire to strengthen the drug laws. The drug laws have been loosening you might say, becoming more relaxed about 20 years. And mandatory minimum sentences have been eliminated. Various things have happened that were unraveling what had taken place before.

Now what was happening was that these laws were being put back into place and actually the Republicans and Democrats seeing this as a tremendous, dangerous issue vied with one another as to all the ways that they were going to help control drugs. In 1986 you started to have the re-imposition of mandatory minimum sentences and then in 1988, two years later, you had a new anti-drug abuse act, which was even more severe than the previous one and this introduced the death penalty for what were called "drug kingpins" and so on. So both parties realized that if either one of them were seen as soft on drugs it would be extremely bad for them in the elections.

It is very difficult for a politician to indicate softness or weakness on drugs. The politicians are afraid to say anything and debate is stifled because you have these two extremes. The drug issue is so polarized that it is difficult to have anything in the middle and because each side feels that they're fighting for their deepest beliefs about themselves and society, and they aren't about to give up easily. So, you can see how difficult it is to strike a happy medium between two extremes.

Interviewer

What are the polls saying now about what Americans are really thinking?

Dr. David Musto

I think that Americans are still very much opposed to the legalization of drugs, from what they understand that to be. And at the same time, there is some indication that people feel that perhaps the penalties for some things are too severe. For example, the penalties for crack are really quite horrendous compared to cocaine, of course crack is cocaine but ...

Interviewer

How about marijuana?

Dr. David Musto

It varies I think from where you live in the country. There are parts of the country in which people would favor essentially the decriminalization of marijuana, and there are other places in which they are very much opposed to it. I think that probably the general consensus is still against marijuana, but there has been quite a development of people feeling that it isn't such a big issue and maybe should be dealt with less dramatically than, let's say, heroin or cocaine.

Interviewer

Marijuana as a "gateway drug"—this is really part of the larger debate too.

Dr. David Musto

In a way marijuana is a gateway drug or alcohol can be a gateway drug, because a lot of people use them and then some of those go onto something else. And in that way, yes, it does precede and it's like the gateway drug. On the other hand, you can't say that everybody who tries alcohol or everybody who tries marijuana then goes on to these other drugs. It pretty much depends on how you feel about this situation. And again, it goes back to how you think things ought to be organized and how they ought to be perceived and the same evidence is seen by one person as proof it isn't a gateway drug and to someone else it settles it that it is.

And one point I wanted to make is that when people are enthusiastic about drugs, and I'd have to go back and read some of the things ... what people said in the 60s because it's hard to believe it now that they believe some of these statements about how marijuana was going to completely change our consciousness and we're all going to move into a new world and so on, or how the insight of LSD, this insight into reality would change everything, these things haven't happened.

The enthusiasm for drugs ... there's a lot of fantasy involved and very little perception of any of the dangers. Only as time goes on and people either become bored with the drugs or they don't do what they're supposed to and they start seeing the bad effects, that people start turning against them. So, in a way, the turning against drugs is more based on experience than the enthusiasm, initially, which is based upon hope as to what the drugs are going to do, and that ... you have to keep in mind when you're talking about these trends.

One of the things that happens though is that it's very hard to convey to the next generation a balanced view that was achieved with great difficulty by the previous generation. That is why so much of the language about drugs is scare language because the thought is we have to instill into a new generation what we've learned. And yet, as we've seen, scare language is sort of self-defeating oftentimes, because it is so exaggerated that it's unreal. You really don't convey anything accurately and what you do is you set yourself up for a disappointment again when people become exposed and they don't, let's say, drop dead from trying that particular substance.

So we have to be very careful how you warn people against drugs that you don't succumb to the absolutely normal temptation to follow the Anslinger style of enormous exaggeration because it in the long run backfires.

I'll give you one example. In 1928 there was a national competition to suggest the way in which we could improve prohibition and make it work. And when I went through the Anslinger papers I came across his submission. He actually sat down and wrote out and submitted it ... [his] whole idea was mandatory minimum sentences for people who drank beer once. Now his view was you'd only have to really put a number of people away for drinking beer once and then a lot of people wouldn't drink beer at all and therefore this was the solution.

So he started off life with the notion that severe penalties have tremendous deterrent effect and they're very worth it. And I think that he ended up with a very different estimate of the power of laws and law enforcement to simply stop drug abuse. And I think that's probably where he would be today. He would still be anti-drug, he would still favor tough law enforcement, but I don't think that he would have, what I call, the kind of naive faith that simply passing horrendous laws is going to cause the drug problem to go away.

Reprinted wiht permission. Interview with Dr. David Musto from *Frontline*, "Busted: America's War on Marijuana" website (http://www.pbs.org/wgbh/pages/frontline/shows/dope/interview/musto.html)

Dr. Musto (1936- 2010), was a professor of child psychiatry in the Child Study Center at the Yale School of Medicine and a professor of the history of medicine. Dr. Musto's book T*he American Disease: Origins of Narcotic Control* (1973) offered a comprehensive account of drug use and government drug policy from the 1860s to the present day. The book was reissued in an expanded edition in 1987 and again in 1999. Dr. Musto was named a consultant to the White House on drug control policy in 1973, and in 1978 he was appointed to the White House Strategy Council on Drug Abuse.

Dr. Musto attended the University of Washington, received a bachelor's degree in classics and a medical degree. He studied the history of science and medicine at Yale and was awarded a master's degree there in 1961.

After completing an internship at Pennsylvania Hospital in Philadelphia and a psychiatric residency at Yale University Medical Center, he was named a special assistant to the director of the National Institute of Mental Health in Bethesda, Md. He also taught for a year at Johns Hopkins University before joining the Child Study Center at Yale in 1969.

He went on to write, with Pamela Korsmeyer, *The Quest for Drug Control*, and edited *One Hundred Years of Heroin* and *Drugs In America: A Documentary History*.

STUART GITLOW MD MPH MBA
President, American Society of Addiction Medicine
New York, N.Y.

The Arguments for Legalization

Marijuana is a plant containing over 400 different chemical compounds, some of which are psychoactive. When combusted and smoked, the number of chemical compounds increases. The psychoactive properties of marijuana, whether smoked or ingested, lead to a desire by some to use the plant for the purposes of intoxication.

Marijuana is not an approved medication, does not come in specific dosages or concentrations, and cannot be prescribed. However, there is anecdotal evidence which suggests that some component or components of marijuana may be useful for patients with chronic pain, side-effects of chemotherapy, and with varying symptoms secondary to HIV infection. In no case have any double-blind placebo-controlled trials demonstrated objectively measurable benefits from the whole plant, either for these purposes or for any medical application.

Use of marijuana carries certain known risks, but the

precise extent of these risks is still uncertain, just as remains the precise extent of any benefits. There is a specific risk of addictive disease, with the greater risks being associated with younger age at onset of use. There is a risk of developing mental health disorders, with psychosis being the most concerning. There is a risk, again particularly in younger individuals, of neuropsychological alterations, with concentration, focus, and attention dropping as would related performance and productivity.

So here we have a plant with no certain benefit to the vast majority who would utilize the substance, and possible benefit to the few who would use it to address certain infrequently occurring medical conditions. We have a plant with known risk that is higher for youth than for adults, just as the risks of alcohol and tobacco are higher for our younger population. We also have, importantly, a society that frequently looks to mind-altering chemicals as a way of entertaining itself. This is true to such an extent that such use represents the leading cause of preventable morbidity, disability, loss of productivity, and mortality.

Within this context, we have a societal push for a third legal psychoactive substance, one that would be added to the already-present burden of alcohol and tobacco. There are several arguments offered for legalization:

The libertarian argument in which each individual should have the right to choose for him or herself whether to take a risk by pursuing certain activities. This argument was utilized in opposition to motorcycle helmet and seat belt laws, but was ultimately quashed by the argument that the greater good to the public outweighed the individual right to choose. This argument is one of a continuum, as we clearly could outlaw downhill skiing, mountain climbing, extreme sports, and other activities that carry risk if we took the argument to its extreme. In this case, we must weigh the overall cost to society, taking into consideration overall loss of productivity, economic damages such as increased healthcare costs, and evidence from tobacco and alcohol that tax-generated revenue is insufficient to offset the gross expenses from the economic damage. We must also take into consideration the benefit that one might theoretically gain; that is, are the intoxicating effects of marijuana different experientially from the alleged benefit of having the wind running through one's hair while riding a motorcycle sans helmet?

The medical argument in which legalization would permit marijuana to be available to those for whom the drug might have medical benefits. In fact, at this writing, there already is a legal form of a marijuana component in the readily available prescription medication, Marinol. Further research is necessary to determine if other components of marijuana offer benefit, at which point those components could be synthesized, packaged in specific doses, and made available by prescription or over-the-counter as called for by associated risks and benefits. The legalization of the plant itself is not necessary to achieve the goal of having medicinal applications for the plant's components. Further, even the anecdotal experience indicates that the medical applications for marijuana components would be of value to only a tiny percentage of the public.

The logical argument in which one states that marijuana is safer than alcohol, and since alcohol is legal, marijuana should be as well. This argument is often based on a statement that one is highly unlikely to overdose and die from marijuana use. Of course, one is equally unlikely to overdose and die from nicotine use while smoking. The dangers of smoking tobacco lie in its likelihood of causing morbidity and mortality over decades of use, not over days of use. But again, one could then state that marijuana is safer than tobacco, and since tobacco is legal, marijuana should be as well. We would then move to a two-wrongs-don't-make-a-right response. Just because the leading cause of death in our society is legal doesn't mean we should add an additional burden of illness. The logic could also be used, with equal weight, to say: Marijuana is safer than tobacco, and since marijuana is illegal, tobacco should be as well. Ultimately, though, this is not a game of comparisons; we know a great deal more now than we did when tobacco was industrialized, and putting the tobacco genie back in the bottle would be far more difficult than would stopping the genie from coming out in the first place.

The risk:benefit argument in which proponents of legalization state that there are no certain risks but certain recreational benefits for marijuana use. This is at the heart of the actual argument, since the majority of marijuana proponents want marijuana not for its purported medicinal application but simply for the recreational aspects of getting intoxicated from use. These proponents do not perceive risk because they themselves have not experienced any negative outcomes. This is equivalent to the 20 year old who has been smoking tobacco for five years, who has no obvious difficulties as a result, and only on reaching 45 and experiencing shortness of breath or a persistent cough does he start to recognize what cards he has dealt himself. The proponent does not care that a minority become addicted because he either is not addicted himself or does not recognize his own addiction. He does not care that a small percentage end up with mental disorders because he does not have a mental disorder. And he does not care that drivers in car accidents have a higher likelihood of marijuana use history than do drivers who have not had car accidents. What he does care about is that he sees marijuana use as providing entertainment through its intoxicating effects, and that there are therefore benefits associated with its use.

The decriminalization argument. This is actually a red herring as decriminalizing use, or possession of small amounts, of marijuana is not equivalent to legalization and a resultant industrialization of farming, packaging, and distributing. If the debate is about whether there are too many marijuana users in jail, then it's not a legalization debate.

The research argument. This is an argument stating that marijuana needs to be legalized for proper research to take place. Again, though, this is a red herring as there are numerous techniques short of legalization that could be utilized to ease the path for appropriate research to take place.

The historic argument: Because marijuana has been used

in its raw form for many years, legalization proponents have argued that research would already have demonstrated significant risks were any present. This fails to take into consideration two important variables. First, marijuana has been altered over the years to a form that generally is much stronger with respect to psychoactive properties than it was only a few decades ago. A study of direct effects or long-term impact of 1970s marijuana would not likely prove applicable to 2010s marijuana. Secondly, research typically requires at least some information regarding dose and frequency if it is to demonstrate related outcomes. Unfortunately, one person's joint, blunt, and bowl may differ significantly from another's. Strains of marijuana vary widely in terms of chemical composition and strengths. Further, unlike tobacco, where users tend to have a consistent dose on a daily basis over many years, marijuana users have historically not generally experienced that degree of consistency. And finally, researchers would argue that indeed there have already been demonstrated several significant risks.

The NIMBY argument: Physicians in states that have legalized some form of dispensed marijuana for medicinal purposes have, in some cases, argued for legalization of marijuana. The goal in these cases is the elimination of physicians being used as a gatekeeper for what is perceived in most cases as being non-medical use of an intoxicant.

The fiscal argument in which state legislators are led to believe that revenue from taxation of legal marijuana will lead to an improved bottom line for their state. They ignore the fact that such taxation has not only not worked in this manner for tobacco or alcohol, but rather that those two legal drugs have cost their states approximately tenfold more than the revenues brought in. Increased costs in the case of marijuana would come not only in regulatory oversight costs, but more importantly in health and disability costs. Lost productivity, driving accidents, disability, hospitalization and emergency room visits for acute and chronic addictive substance use and its sequelae: all would take their toll in terms of increasing public costs. The costs will initially lag behind the revenue; this will have the unfortunate effect of leading pundits to initially argue that taxation of marijuana is a winning game for states.

The argument stating, "Everyone uses marijuana anyway, and therefore legalization will not result in any significant increase in use." Untrue. It has been well demonstrated that use of marijuana rises as perception of risk falls. Legalization serves to demonstrate to the public that marijuana has low risk, something guaranteed to lead to increased utilization. We have been down this path before with alcohol. Per capita use of alcohol fell dramatically and precipitously when Prohibition was instituted, and rose dramatically in the years after Prohibition ended. There are, in fact, many who obey the law, and who have not used marijuana simply because such use is illegal.

At the end of the day, all of the arguments for legalization of marijuana have yet to be convincing. The best argument is indeed the one which often goes unspoken: some individuals simply want the right to get stoned, free of potential legal consequences, and without concern as to whether that right would carry a likelihood of harm for either themselves or others. Were we not living in a society where we each have responsibility for one another's health and welfare, perhaps such an argument would rule the day.

Stuart Gitlow, MD MPH MBA is Executive Director of the Annenberg Physician Training Program in Addictive Disease at Mount Sinai School of Medicine in New York, NY, which he started in 2005 to ensure medical student access to training that stimulates them to develop and maintain interest in working with patients with addiction. Now dividing his time between a clinical addiction medicine practice in New England and academic work in New York, Dr Gitlow is on the faculty of both Dartmouth College in Hanover, NH, and Mount Sinai School of Medicine. He obtained his MD at Mount Sinai School of Medicine, his psychiatric and public health training at University of Pittsburgh, PA, and a forensic psychiatry fellowship at Harvard University in Boston, MA. Dr Gitlow serves as Chair of the AMA's Council on Science and Public Health. He is President of the American Society of Addiction Medicine and its delegate to the AMA. Dr Gitlow formerly produced both Health Channel and ABC programming at America Online. Member SAM Science Advisory Board USA.

AMY J. PORATH-WALLER, PH.D., JONATHAN E. BROWN, PH.D., AARIN P. FRIGON, M.A., CHRP, HEATHER CLARK, M.A.
Canadian Centre on Substance Abuse
Ottawa, Ontario

What Canadian Youth Think about Cannabis, Report in Short, 2013

For more than 25 years, the Canadian Centre on Substance Abuse (CCSA) has provided national leadership and advanced solutions to address alcohol—and other drug-related harm. Together with its partners, the Centre is working to improve the health and safety of Canadians by nurturing a knowledge exchange environment, where research guides policy and evidence-informed actions enhance effectiveness in the field.

The Issue

Canadian youth are the top users of cannabis in the developed world.[1] Despite a decrease in cannabis use among youth in recent years,[2] cannabis remains the most commonly used illegal drug among Canadian youth, 15–24 years of age.[3] In fact, the number of youth who have used cannabis within the last year is currently three times higher than that of adults aged 25 years and older (21.6% vs. 6.7%).[3] In some Canadian jurisdictions, approximately 50% of grade 12 students have reported consuming cannabis within the last year.[4]

Although cannabis can produce feelings of euphoria and relaxation, its use can lead to negative consequences. Short-term use can cause difficulties in brain functions such as memory, perception of time, coordination and balance.[5] These effects can lead to injuries or car crashes when driving.[6] In addition to health and safety concerns, youth substance abuse can also lead to difficulties at school and problems with relationships and the law.[7]

Adolescents are particularly at risk for cannabis related harms since their brains are undergoing rapid and extensive development. Research tells us that chronic cannabis use is associated with memory, thinking and attention difficulties, particularly among those who began using cannabis in early adolescence.[8] Chronic use might also increase the risk of psychosis, depression and anxiety, in addition to respiratory conditions and possibly lung cancer.[9,10,11,12]

Although there is an increasing amount of knowledge related to the harms linked to cannabis use, we know little about what youth think about the drug and what influences their decisions to use it. To begin addressing this knowledge gap the Canadian Centre on Substance Abuse (CCSA) conducted a study to examine these perceptions. Highlights of the full report are described below.

Description of the Study

The purpose of the study was to increase our understanding of youth perceptions about cannabis use in order to inform the development of initiatives to prevent youth cannabis use and abuse. Youth were asked to describe how their peers' decisions to use cannabis were influenced by family, other youth, community, the law and the medical use of cannabis. Seventy-six youth, aged 14 to 19 years, participated in one of 10 in-person or two online focus groups conducted in five urban and rural Canadian locations. Thirty-eight percent of participants were female. Sixty-two percent of the youth had used cannabis in the past and approximately half of these respondents indicated they had used it within the last 24 hours.

Key Findings

Influences for Smoking and Not Smoking Cannabis

Parents, siblings and friends appear to influence decisions by young people to use cannabis. Youth in the study mentioned that some parents do not make their position on cannabis use clear. Other parents, it was felt, use cannabis with their kids or are disengaged from their children's lives. Peer pressure, social connectedness to peers and the drug's perceived popularity and availability were also mentioned as factors influencing use. In fact, youth held a common belief that "everyone smokes weed" and perceived that not using cannabis is abnormal:

" … people who aren't trying marijuana … are not standing up because they don't want to [be] looked down upon … everyone is just too scared."

Concerns about health risks, poor academic performance and the negative impacts on family relationships were also felt to prevent youth from using cannabis. Interestingly, trouble with the law was not mentioned as a factor deterring use.

Perceived Positive and Negative Effects of Cannabis

Youth in the study discussed perceived positive effects more often than negative effects. These included the drug's ability to help youth focus, relax, sleep, be less violent and improve creativity, as well as how it can purify your system or cure cancer:

"For me, I'm thinking about for my health. … Because I smoke two pack of cigarettes a day. A cigarette gives you cancer, but the weed cover it. It going to clean it up."

Perceived negative effects included developing dependency, losing focus, becoming lazy, developing lung and heart conditions, and increasing criminality. Participants perceived cannabis to affect each person differently, and negative effects, including long-term changes in chronic users, were attributed to the individual and not cannabis itself.

Cannabis as Natural and Safe, and Not a Drug

Many youth did not consider cannabis to be a drug. When asked why, responses included that it was natural (not man-made), safe and non-addictive, and that it reduced violent tendencies and did not change the user's perception of reality, unlike harder drugs.

"I don't look at weed as a drug. I just look at it as another thing you smoke, like a cigarette."

It was widely felt cannabis is much safer than alcohol and tobacco. Participants preferred the term "smoking weed" to "using cannabis," given that the term "using" was associated with addiction to harder drugs.

Cannabis and Driving

A number of the youth believed that cannabis is safe and makes people better drivers by increasing their focus. Drunk driving was seen as being much more dangerous than driving under the influence of cannabis. In contrast, others felt that using cannabis while driving is dangerous and constitutes impaired driving. However, even those opposed to using cannabis and driving stated that it is not as dangerous as drunk driving.

" … it started to make me more cautious and I started to pay more attention to the roads, signs and everything that's going on around me."

Legality of Cannabis

Participants were confused about the legality of cannabis. Some felt cannabis was legal depending on age and the amount in your possession. It appeared that the inconsistent reactions of police to cannabis and the legality of medical marijuana were, in part, leading to the confusion.

"After 19 you are allowed to have a little on you, no more than 1.5, I think. … You're allowed, you can use a little bit. But if they catch you with a pound you're screwed."

Perceptions of Effective Prevention Approaches

In the study youth argued that general information about drugs presented using scare tactics is an ineffective approach to prevention. They suggested that effective approaches would involve providing more fact-based information at an earlier age, providing more content relating specifically to cannabis (and not all drugs) and using approaches that are aimed at reducing the harms of using cannabis, rather than focusing on abstinence. "They just make stupid ... commercials that everyone is like, that's not what happens."

Participants also suggested that to be effective prevention efforts should ensure that those who deliver prevention messages have an ability to connect with youth, as well as have first-hand experience with the drug.

Implications

Although based on a small sample size, the findings of this study highlight the complexity surrounding the use of cannabis by youth in Canada and point to the challenges associated with preventing its use and misuse. Canadian youth appear confused with what they perceive as the current mixed messaging they receive about this illicit drug. The study underscores the need for a coordinated, comprehensive, factual and consistent approach specific to preventing cannabis use and abuse. Such prevention efforts need to reflect the lived reality of Canadian youth and address existing misperceptions by clearly communicating what we know about cannabis—both harms and benefits—and what information is still emerging.

Consideration should also be given to creating supportive environments in the home, school and community that do not normalize the use of cannabis, but instead redefine social norms. This change would include building awareness that the majority of youth do not use cannabis. Focusing awareness on the impact of cannabis on brain development could also provide a fact-based way to encourage dialogue. The influence of peers, parents and family in decisions to use or not use cannabis points to the importance of their involvement in prevention and encouraging healthy lifestyles.

When asked directly, youth identified several key considerations they thought would be helpful for cannabis-related prevention efforts. These included increasing content specific to cannabis in prevention programs and materials, delivering prevention efforts at a much earlier age, ensuring those delivering the prevention message have credibility with youth and selecting approaches aimed at reducing the harms associated with cannabis use.

....

References

1 UNICEF Office of Research (2013). Child well-being in rich countries: A comparative overview, *Innocenti Report Card 11*, UNICEF Office of Research, Florence.

2 Although cannabis is the illegal drug most commonly used by youth, its use in recent years has decreased. According to the 2011 Canadian Alcohol and Drug Use Monitoring Survey (CADUMS), 37% of youth in 2004 reported using cannabis in the past year compared to 21.6% in 2011.

3 Health Canada. (2012). Canadian Alcohol and Drug Use Monitoring Survey: Summary of results for 2011.

4 Young, M.M., Saewyc, E., Boak, A., Jahrig, J., Anderson, B., Doiron, Y., Taylor, S., Pica, L., Laprise, P., and Clark, H. (2011). *Cross-Canada report on student alcohol and drug use: Technical report*. Ottawa, ON: Canadian Centre on Substance Abuse.

5 Porath-Waller, A.J. (2013). *Clearing the smoke on cannabis: Highlights.* Ottawa, ON: Canadian Centre on Substance Abuse.

6 Asbridge, M., Hayden, J.A., & Cartwright, J.L. (2012). Acute cannabis consumption and motor vehicle collision risk: systematic review of observational studies and meta-analysis. *British Medical Journal, 344, e536.*

7 Canadian Centre on Substance Abuse and Ontario Centre of Excellence for Child and Youth Mental Health. (2013). *When mental health and substance abuse problems collide*. Ottawa: ON: Authors.

8 Porath-Waller, A.J. (2009a). *Clearing the smoke on cannabis: Chronic use and cognitive functioning and mental health*. Ottawa, ON: Canadian Centre on Substance Abuse.

9 Beirness, D.J., & Porath-Waller, A.J. (2009). *Clearing the smoke on cannabis: Cannabis use and driving*. Ottawa, ON: Canadian Centre on Substance Abuse.

10 Diplock, J., & Plecas, D. (2009). *Clearing the smoke on cannabis: Respiratory effects of cannabis smoking*. Ottawa, ON: Canadian Centre on Substance Abuse.

11 Kalant, H., & Porath-Waller, A.J. (2012). *Clearing the smoke on cannabis: Medical use of cannabis and cannabinoids*. Ottawa, ON: Canadian Centre on Substance Abuse.

12 Porath-Waller, A.J. (2009b). *Clearing the smoke on cannabis: Maternal cannabis use during pregnancy*. Ottawa, ON: Canadian Centre on Substance Abuse.

What Canadian Youth Think about Cannabis: Report in Short, 2013, reproduced with permission from the Canadian Centre on Substance Abuse. This research and report were made possible through a financial contribution from Health Canada's Drug Strategy Community Initiatives Fund, however the views expressed herein do not necessarily reflect the views of Health Canada.

For further information, consult the full report, *What Canadian Youth Think about Cannabis: Technical Report, 2013 (http://www.ccsa.ca/Resource%20 Library/CCSA-What-Canadian-Youth-Think-about-Cannabis-2013-en.pdf)*

JO MCGUIRE

What Are the Costs Associated with Marijuana Legalization?

An employer who takes the view that Friday night use of marijuana is none of his concern will begin to see ramifications when impairment on Monday morning endangers workplace safety. As marijuana legalization surges across our nation, many of us view it as an inevitable tidal wave of unquestioning change that we must consider the new cultural norm. The prevailing mindset seems to be that "everyone wants it." However, the simple fact that the marijuana lobby has a brilliant marketing strategy of social norming does not mean that everyone wants marijuana legalization, nor does it indicate that our responses to this issue are coming from an informed point of view.

Common sense has employers concerned about the impacts of impairment in the workplace, but the pressures and threats that using marijuana is the constitutional right of the employee causes entire corporations to consider backing down from drug-free workplace policies that help ensure public health and safety. Common sense would also have parents and school personnel recognizing the harm to young people, but the constant thrum that marijuana is harmless (and even ... good medicine) has many authority figures looking the other way when it comes to teen marijuana use because we are prone to believe everyone is doing it.

In the same vein of thought that draws these conclusions, we also hear that marijuana should be viewed the same way as alcohol, which is socially acceptable for adults, yet we would never consider it appropriate to use alcohol in a way that negatively impacts the workplace or allow kids to use alcohol with abandon.

According to The Economic Costs of Alcohol Abuse report, alcoholism costs U.S. employers 500 million lost work days per year (NIDA, 2000). The cost of alcohol abuse in the United States is at least $185 billion annually. In other words, for every dollar we bring in, we spend ten. Why are we holding this up as a revenue model?

It has been said that by regulating marijuana like alcohol, teen use will decrease; but taking into account that in 2009 more than 70 percent of teens 18 years and under had experienced drinking alcohol, it does not seem possible that treating marijuana as alcohol will result in less use by teens (NIH, 2009). When adolescents use marijuana regularly, they can experience a lasting 6-8 point I.Q. reduction that, for most people, drops them significantly for potentially completing their education and gaining substantial future employment (Meier, et al., 2012).

Treating marijuana the same as alcohol is impossible for several reasons. The potency and serving suggestions for marijuana cannot be standardized in the same way regulatory authorities have measured alcohol, due to lack of uniform measurement techniques. Additionally, there are no measurements for marijuana impairment that relate across the board to how we understand alcohol impairment. A simple breath alcohol test allows us to know the immediate blood-alcohol ratio impacting the subject's brain, where no such standard exists for marijuana.

To be exact, no such measurement will be ready for years to come.

Current options allow for employers, law enforcement officers, or medical personnel to simply find marijuana present in the subject's system. Metabolized rates of THC (the psychoactive component of marijuana) vary widely based on each individual's body type. However, impairment cannot be measured by a simple screening test.

Where alcohol impairment rates are fairly standard, marijuana impairment rates are wildly unpredictable. As commercialized marijuana products continue to be refined and enhanced, allowing for soaring levels of THC that are commonly 10-20 times more potent than in previous decades, some users report effects of acute impairment lasting for days after use. Therefore, an employer who takes the view that Friday night use of marijuana is none of his concern will begin to see ramifications when impairment on Monday morning endangers workplace safety.

Zero Tolerance Supports Public Safety

These are just a few of the reasons it remains imperative for employers to maintain thorough and consistent screening practices in order to strengthen Safe and Drug-Free Workplace stances. As screening becomes more advanced through techniques such as oral swabbing, which allows for shorter detection time with THC, sending strong messages that impairment in the workplace will not be tolerated is both public safety and fiscally responsible.

While the marijuana industry does project billions of dollars streaming into the economy through tax revenues, pols and pundits alike fail to attempt to calculate cost load (Fairchild, 2013). Here are some important things we must consider:

A federal report on workplace drug testing by SAMHSA states that employees using marijuana cause 55 percent more accidents than those who do not, and positive drug tests showing THC in the employee's system verifies 85 percent more on-the-job injuries by marijuana users (Autry, 1998). This same report lists increased absenteeism and loss of work productivity as additional costs to the U.S. employer. While the National Drug Intelligence Center reports that substance abuse costs this country upwards of $193 billion each year, these costs are limited in scope and do not include the costs of associated destructive behaviors, such as child abuse or domestic violence (National Drug Intelligence Center, 2011).

Regardless of what the commercialization proponents say in paid advertising campaigns, marijuana does produce a dependence that requires addiction recovery and treatment. Data sets from the National Survey on Drug Use and Health from 2012 show admissions to addiction treatment facilities document marijuana as the second-highest reason for treatment—directly behind alcohol (NSDUH, 2014). The Partnership for Drug-Free Kids states that 23.5 million Americans are addicted to alcohol and drugs, which amounts to one in every 10 people over the age of 12 (Join Together, 2010). The financial burden of addiction and recovery treatment has yet to be fully addressed in efforts for national health care reform, but one thing we do know is that costs are staggeringly out of control.

According to an article in Annals of Emergency Medicine, those states that began allowing marijuana for medical use before 2005 saw calls to poison control centers for children accidentally exposed to marijuana triple. In states that have not permitted marijuana for medical use, there were no incidents (Wang, 2014). In Colorado, where recreational marijuana has been permitted, cases of child poisonings have risen significantly with at least two cases of small children requiring intubation to continue breathing. Cannabis related emergency hospital admission rates overall have been rising sharply in the United States, according to the Drug Abuse Warning Network (DAWN), which shows emergency department admissions rose from 16,251 in 1991 to more than 461,028 in 2012 (SAM HSA, 2013). Marijuana-related admissions to hospital emergency rooms account for more than all other drugs combined.

While we hear repeatedly that marijuana is "safe," we desperately need a definition of what entails "safety" when emergency rooms are burdened with marijuana-related health issues.

Where marijuana for medical use has been touted as a revenue stream, an audit of the Colorado system (touted as the world's finest regulatory implementation) showed heavy financial losses to the point of operating at a deficit with violations of the regulatory system rampant (Ray, 2013). This has not seemed to be a large-scale consideration as we look through the lenses of dollar signs with recreational marijuana.

Colorado law enforcement is continually strapped to cover costs associated with road-side drug testing when alcohol is not the culprit of an impaired driver. To date, the framework for marijuana regulation does not include reimbursement to local or statewide jurisdictions for expenditures on trained Drug Recognition Experts, blood tests, or court costs associated with traffic offenses. These are losses suffered at the taxpayers' expense.

Problems Associated with Legalization

In a compiled report by Dr. Bertha Madras of the Harvard Medical School's Department of Psychiatry, marijuana use disorder is associated with higher mortality. It has lasting adverse effects on the future of young adults through increases of anxiety, panic, depression, psychotic symptoms, cognitive losses, and neuropsychological decline and causes various adverse health effects, such as psychosis (Madras, 2012). Our nation's Mental Health Parity Act has not been fully implemented to address the scope of mental health issues that are exacerbated by marijuana use, rather than clinical treatment.

Questions still left unanswered would be the impact of second-hand marijuana smoke to children and family members and costs related to associated illnesses. Much less the fact that smoking marijuana puts the user at similar, if not greater, risks associated with tobacco. The California Office of Environmental Health Hazards' assessment on the carcinogenicity of marijuana smoke states, "[s]tudies reporting results for direct marijuana smoking have observed statistically significant associations with cancers of the lung, head and neck, bladder, brain, and testis. The strongest evidence of a causal association was for head and neck cancer, with two of four studies reporting statistically significant associations. The evidence was less strong but suggestive for lung cancer, with one of three studies conducted in populations that did not mix marijuana and tobacco reporting a significant association. Suggestive evidence also was seen for bladder cancer, with one of two studies reporting a significant association. For brain and testicular cancers, the single studies conducted of each of these endpoints reported significant associations" (Tomar PhD, Beaumont PhD, & Ysieh PhD, 2009).

There are far more questions and problems associated with the legalization of marijuana (with no compelling medical evidence to remove it as a Federally Controlled Schedule 1 Substance) than there are good solutions at this point. While it is clear that thoughtful dialogue should take place in order to learn more and formulate positive strategies, fast-tracking a recreational drug to legal status through a ruse of impossible regulatory ideologies will prove irresponsible and costly. Exact figures of societal costs will not be known for many years to come, if they are ever able to be truly calculated, but we must keep the whole spectrum of issues pertaining to marijuana at the forefront of our decision and policy-making efforts.

....

References

1. Autry, J. H. (1998). Testimony on Federal Workplace Drug Testing. Washington D.C.: SAMHSA.
2. Fairchild, C. (2013, April 20). Legalizing Marijuana Would Generate Billions in Additional Tax Revenue Annually. Retrieved July 15, 2014, from Huffington Post: http://www.huffingtonpost.com/2013/04/20/legalizing-marijuana-tax revenue_n_3102003.html
3. Join Together. (2010, September 28). New Data Show Millions of Americans with Alcohol and Drug Addiction Could Benefit from Health Care. Retrieved July
15, 2014, from Drug Free America: http://www.drugfree.org/new-data-show millions-of-americans-with-alcohol-and-drug-addiction-could-benefit-from health-care-r/
4. Madras, B. P. (2012). What the Latest Top Cannabis Research Tells Us. Retrieved July 15, 2014, from drthurstone.com: http://drthurstone.com/what latest-top-cannabis-research-tells-us/
5. Meier, M., Caspi, A., Ambler, A., Keefe, R., McDonald, K., Ward, A., et al. (2012). Persistent Cannabis Users Show Neuropsychological Decline from Child hood to Midlife. Durham: PNAIS.
6. National Drug Intelligence Center. (2011). The Economic Impact of Illicit Drug Use on American Society. Washington D.C.: U.S. Department of Justice.

Reprinted with permission. *Occupational Health and Safety*, September 1, 2014.

While serving as the director for Compliance and Corporate Training in the field of workplace drug and alcohol testing, **Jo McGuire** was appointed to serve on the Governor's Task Force that was convened to recommend a legislative framework for the regulation of marijuana in Colorado. She served in this capacity as part of the Taxation, Banking and Civil Law work group and lent her expertise in the form of recommendations for drug and alcohol testing in the workplace. She serves on the Board of Directors for the Drug and Alcohol Testing Industry Association and co-chairs the International Marijuana Education Committee with the Board Chairman, Phil Dubois. Her current project, called "Of Substance Media," will provide a clearinghouse of information and scientific, evidence-based research that will aid in countering the harmful effects of addictive and illicit substances.

DAVID BERNER
Executive Director, Drug Prevention Network of Canada
Therapist, Orchard Recovery Centre
Vancouver, B.C.

The Pot Kids

Every week for several years now, I work with teens who have already slipped down the rabbit hole. Look up "dazed and confused" and their passport photos come up.

These kids have had no role models or lousy role models. They have latched on to the first person of any strength who happens to be standing near them. Unfortunately, that character is usually the neighbourhood dope dealer. The kids are lazy, undisciplined, without focus or purpose. Their goals are all immediate gratification and survival. Some are brash, but most are sullen and shy. My first job is to create a sense of safety and that old bugaboo, trust. Slowly, ever so painfully slowly, we draw these kids into real conversation. (All the while taking care of basics like food and sleep and recreation and a bit of fun.) Most of these youngsters can begin to see fairly soon the trauma they have experienced and pushed beneath the surface and the near fatal bad choices they've been making.That'll happen when you have little self-belief and no one else around you seems to give you value as well.

Unbelievably, so many of these teens and early twenties kids get it. Often, it takes less than a month, a few weeks, for them to start to return to life, to do two really important things that they haven't done in a while - laugh and think! Often, we are able to bring their parents and siblings into the picture and wade through those mine fields and begin to find some sense, and some sense of love.

David Berner

Adam started smoking marijuana when he was eight.

Now he is 32 and he is using crystal meth (or crack cocaine or heroin and certainly alcohol). We can help him get off his current drug of choice; that's easy. A day or two of small fuss and bother and it's over. But when he returns after 28 or 42 days to what passes for his normal life away from the intensity, camaraderie and focus of the treatment centre regime, he will consider his pot smoking 'regular.' What's the problem? This is like breathing or going to the bathroom. Isn't this what everyone does? Huh? Pot will be in his circle of expectations, a given, axiomatic.

To complicate matters, Adam has never worked a day in his life. He has no skill sets or work ethic or even the simplest notions of getting up, showering, eating breakfast and getting to the office, plant or work site on time. If there's an alarm clock in the house, he hasn't met it yet. When you ask him or Janine in group what they do, they giggle and look around the room in a kind of challenging bemusement. They don't understand the question. Do? What do you mean, do? A man is 32 or a woman is 26 and they have no concept of work, let alone vagaries like accomplishment and goals. Adam and Janine have survived by selling small amounts of drugs, by lying and cheating and by manipulating their parents and siblings and other family members into paying the bills. Occasionally they rent out their body parts by the half hour.

These young men and women belong to no one special socio-economic group. They are rich and poor. They have parents who are monsters and parents who are saints and parents who are like all of the rest of us in between. Their color, race, religion and sexual orientation cover all the spectra. Addictions are blind to all these troublesome details.

Already you are saying, well, this is a shame. We're sorry to learn that you meet people like this from time to time.

No.

Here's the scoop. There are hundreds of thousands of young men and women like Adam and Janine in every town and city across North America. They are The New Addict.

The New Addicts began to show their smiley faces about 30 years ago. Before that, through generations of immigrants and tough times and the new post-war luxuries of fridges and big cars with bench seats, everyone assumed that work was basic. The tall people in the house disappeared all day, and then, over the kitchen table, told all their stories about the indignities and comedies of what happened at this place called 'work.' For all the short people, including those unfortunates who grew up to be addicts and alcoholics, there was a commonly held belief that cleaning up included or concluded with going back into the work force, maybe even realizing a dream or two that had been momentarily sacrificed on the altars of smack or gin.

Now, in the drooping centre of our Unending Abundance and in our Age of Entitlement, we have the New Addict who more than ever is the poster child for complete and total self-indulgence. In group work and in lectures and workshops, these clients and students have embraced the foetal position as their fallback posture. They sit with their feet on the furniture. They suck on candies or coffee or juice. They are old enough to vote, make babies or go to war and they are perennial children stuck firmly in a time long lost.

They expect little of themselves and everything of everyone else. If we are seasoned counselors or therapists, we will cure them, fix them, and slip the magic formula to them under the table. You mean I am supposed to work at this recovery thing? Puleeeese…

The parents and families are often both Controllers and Enablers all at once, first telling their petulant progeny what to do and them rescuing them anyway when they don't follow instructions and land once again in the soup.

Now, let's leave these irksome souls aside for a moment and consider marijuana in general.

We all know good people, productive people, solid citizens

who smoke a joint or two and carry on with a good head and a good heart. I have a friend who is at the top of his field, brilliant and tireless in his contributions, who smokes a joint every night as he's getting into bed. Why do I care? Why should I? Why should you? Seven days a week, this man is completely sober and dedicated to helping others and to increasing the body of knowledge in his area of concern.

Millions of people around the world enjoy wine and vodka and bourbon without becoming cave people. Some people just can't seem to do that. One drink leads to seven and that leads to three days and nights in a row of complete madness. These poor souls are called Alcoholics. If they are lucky, they fall into a meeting of Alcoholics Anonymous or a counselor's office before they kill themselves and six innocent others on the freeway or watch their internal organs fall apart unto death.

Nobody is claiming that marijuana is universally and in every imaginable aspect an evil thing. It may help some sufferers survive otherwise untreatable pain. So some people claim and that's fine with me. (Although the huge numbers of folks now lining up for their so-called medical marijuana suggests that a great many good time Charlies are just looking for an acceptable and legal way to get stoned.)

But there is absolutely no question that, for so many vulnerable young people, marijuana is a gateway drug that leads inevitably to the hell called addiction – addiction to almost any wacky substance that's available.

How do we know this to be so?

Almost as bad as addictions themselves is the current vogue among so-called helpers, authorities and experts to speak in quasi and pseudo-scientific jargon. Everybody and his aunt these days want to pose as a doctor. They urgently seek validation from the community at large. As one comedian famously used to say, "M.D.—Me Doctor."

I have sat in clinical meetings in recovery centres and listened to people with minimal training in anything other than deceptions and dissembling speak as if they were board certified pharmacists. They prattle off the names of exotic pharmaceuticals and how they should be administered to clients without asking for even a moment how is Bob doing or what are we hearing from Jean these days?

One of the favorite phrases such strivers love to bandy about is this choice catch-all: evidence-based. Twelve step programs, for example, are debased because they may not be 'evidence-based.' Really? And what do you say to the literally millions of clean and sober citizens who found their renewed dignity by attending meetings of Alcoholics Anonymous, Cocaine Anonymous and Narcotics Anonymous? Are their living, breathing examples not evidence enough that something appears to be working?

Residential recovery programs are questioned because they often don't have stark statistics on what someone wants to call 'success.' There are some very good reasons for this. We are not measuring cars that work and vacuum cleaners that don't work. We are talking about human beings, complicated and unpredictable. I dare you to handicap people in treatment and put money on the possible winners and losers. The person who seemed for the whole month of treatment to be really engaged falls into the first bar he sees on the way home. The lady who seemed to be staring blankly through every process is now in her second year of sobriety. Go figure.

Say Bill is a heroin addict who now limits himself to a couple of beers on a Friday night. Can we put him in the success column? I would and I'm one of those old-fashioned Neanderthals who strives for and believes entirely in abstinence. Perhaps Darlene is a crack head who now smokes the occasional joint. Not ideal, but who and what is? I've got her listed under 'success.'

So how do we know for sure that these New Addicts actually exist and that they think that marijuana is like furniture—it's always there and it's meant to be used? Where is the 'evidence?' Which scientific journal has proclaimed these truths? Anecdotal evidence is decried as not scientific at all; it's just a good story. But what happens when these stories are all around you, when hundreds and thousands of recovery workers will attest that they are meeting these men and women every day who take pot for granted as part of the landscape to which they are completely entitled?

The central argument of this piece is that the liberalization and normalization of marijuana is dreadfully harmful to our children and to our communities.

Let's ask first why this is happening and second what role does the media play?

The first rule of journalism is 'Follow the Money,' and in

the case of marijuana nothing could be simpler. When pot was declared legal in the state of Washington, people traveled from New York and points beyond to join the celebration. Interviewed on the news, the revelers claimed this was all about freedom of choice. This was a great day for democracy. They are mistaken and deluded. But what would you expect from folks whose main raison d'etre is getting and staying high?

This was, in fact, a great day for capitalism and free markets. Not since the California Gold Rush in the middle of the nineteenth century has there been so much energy, enthusiasm and drift given to one commodity and its apparently limitless potential. Australia's ABC television news crew came to Seattle and assembled a fascinating and chilling documentary called "Cannabis, Inc." One sees, among other things, smart, young Masters of the Universe in slick Boss suits talking about their IPO's being capitalized in the billions of dollars as they prepare their new medical marijuana companies. These amoral bastards were selling pork futures and swamp land in Florida last year. Now, they cloak themselves in some imaginary garb of medical legitimacy and sell pot. Here in Canada, two former big city mayors, one former Provincial Premier, one current senator and a former Member of Parliament have all signed on as board members of similar new pot enterprises. They are all getting on in years and maybe their retirement planning wasn't top notch. Not to worry. Now they will all be set.

The price for their comfort is simple: our children.

The media may be even more culpable in their contribution to this doomed bandwagon than the entrepreneurs themselves. Every single day, every newspaper and telecast includes at least one pot story. These pieces are starkly different from what might have run 10 years ago. Today, grow-ops next door to you and pot shops and pot dispensaries and pot farms and pot licences are spoken of in a manner that says, "This is just normal business, folks. Don't get your shirt in a knot." As public communicators, we are doing everything we can to normalize marijuana, to make it an acceptable part of the landscape. It's just like oranges or skis or baseball caps. National and local news anchors clown and joke and wink at each other on camera when pot is the subject. Hahaha... Isn't it just precious that anyone would care about people using pot today? Hahaha...

The only problem is that this snapshot of reality is a fiction. It is simply not true. If we could ever get the unions or labor relations boards or workers' compensation people to admit it, 90% of the industrial accidents that occur today on work sites have happened because so many of the people on site started their day with a little joint on the way to the job. While China extends its influence to every port and every sovereign country in the world, America and Canada have never been less productive. We spend so much time and energy rallying for the desperately important right to get stoned when and how we choose. Perhaps we might re-direct that energy to building something.

There is a Canadian who spent a few years in an American jail for some offense or other. He calls himself "The Prince of

Pot." When he came home recently, he boasted that he was now smoking 16-20 joints a day. He has been greeted as a hero. Could you please explain to me how a grown man whose entire focus in life is to have no focus, to blot himself out every day, how this person can be seen as a hero. Nelson Mandela is a hero.

Already we are seeing children in Denver hospitals for eating marijuana cookies that have turned out to be toxic. Marijuana shop owners are being robbed and held up and the illegal drug trade hasn't slowed down one beat. And it will not. The criminals are endlessly creative and resourceful. They will always find new and inventive ways to make a rotten buck. That's what they do. That's why they are called criminals. If you have a drug dealer fouling the street in front of your gelato store, don't call the cops. Call the local branch of the Angels; they'll clean up this little problem right smart and thank you for it.

Nobody thinks the War on Drugs has been any kind of success. Nobody wants people thrown in jail for smoking a joint. Somewhere between prohibition and complete resignation to Marijuana Nation lies a movement called SAM, Smart Approaches to Marijuana. Google them and check them out. They're not on anything; but they are onto something and it's good.

And let's go back to where we started, to Adam and Janine, our New Addicts who began their drug-addled lives with marijuana at the age of eight and still think that's as regular as Rice Krispies. As we continue as a misguided, thoughtless society to make pot OK and peachy keen for pretty much everybody all the time, we can only expect millions more young people to be caught in the web of addictions. Soon, thanks to the new decriminalization postures, new legalization laws and broad new acceptance of marijuana as one of God's great gifts, Adam and Janine will have many new friends. Many will graduate to tougher, more toxic and dangerous poisons and to interactions with tougher and more dangerous associates.

I smoked marijuana in my early twenties. It was a lot of dumb fun. I never thought it was a religious experience or a quick way to enlightenment. It was just dumb fun. But sooner or later, we are called upon to leave the things of childhood behind us. People posing as grown-ups who devote all their talents and energies to pot have a serious problem.

A culture that has so little regard for its children that it makes every effort to open the doors to addictions is in serious trouble.

Some rigorous self-examination is in order.

David Berner was the Founder (1967) and Executive Director of Canada's first Residential Treatment Centre for drug addicts and alcoholics. The Foundation continues to thrive and send hundreds of people each year back into the community as clean and sober citizens. Mr. Berner is also an actor, writer and broadcaster. He has compiled a 5-page resume of performances in radio, television, stage and film.

He is a regular contributor to local magazines and websites and last year he published his first book, "ALL THE WAY HOME," chronicling the history and theory of his addictions work.

He is best known for his many years as an enormously popular Radio Talk Show Host on CKNW Radio, and these days you can see him five times a week on his public affairs show on SHAW COMMUNITY TV, CABLE 4.

David conducts therapy, counseling and process groups for several long-established treatment centres on regular basis.

David is the Executive Director of the Drug Prevention Network of Canada.

SAMUEL A. BALL
President and Chief Executive of CASA Columbia University,
and a professor of psychiatry at Yale Medical School

What Science Says About Marijuana

THE MEASURING OF marijuana's addictive potential and consequences against our two most highly profitable, deadly and legal drugs—tobacco and alcohol—as a justification for its legalization seems to me to reflect a terrible cynicism about public health, and it distracts attention from the research findings.

Is it really acceptable for one out of every 10 marijuana users (among adolescents, nearly one of every five) to have a diagnosable disorder? The majority (two-thirds) of adolescent substance abuse treatment admissions involve marijuana as the primary disorder.

Other scientific facts need emphasis separate from their comparison to alcohol and tobacco. Regular marijuana use is associated with cognitive, educational and respiratory problems. It increases risk for other substance and psychiatric diagnoses. Scientific disagreement remains about marijuana as a "gateway" drug; it is not a myth that has been disproved.

Marijuana addiction and withdrawal are considered physical because this potent drug causes significant changes in the brain. Finally, the belief that marijuana addiction and health problems will be managed better by legalization and government regulation has no basis in science or history.

Decisions about the safety of our country's youth should not be made exclusively in the court of public, political and media opinion. I hope the science of marijuana addiction will not be minimized or distorted in this polarizing debate.

Samuel A. Ball is the President and Chief Executive of CASA, Columbia University, and Professor of Psychiatry at Yale Medical School.

HAZELDEN BETTY FORD FOUNDATION

Statement Against Legalization of Marijuana

As THE NATION'S largest nonprofit provider of addiction prevention, treatment and recovery services, the Hazelden Betty Ford Foundation has an important responsibility, and is uniquely qualified, to comment on the effects of marijuana use, which we see every day among the people we serve at our 15 locations around the country.

We know marijuana is dangerous to many users and addictive to some, and that young people are particularly vulnerable. While the debates over legalization continue, many young people view marijuana as less risky, and not surprisingly, more and more of them are smoking marijuana for the first time.

Early use of marijuana is especially troubling. The human brain develops throughout adolescence and well beyond. Marijuana use can harm learning, thinking and memory development and can contribute to mental health issues, not to mention medical problems. We also know the earlier a young person starts to use any mood and mind altering substance, the greater the possibility of developing addiction. One of the recurring themes we hear from the youth we treat is regret—of wasted time, lost opportunities, squandered talent, impaired memory, reduced performance and disinterest in healthy activities.

Expanded social acceptance will almost certainly result in more new users, higher frequency of use among established users and increases in marijuana-associated health and social problems.

Therefore, the Hazelden Betty Ford Foundation opposes any efforts that increase the availability of marijuana and minimize the dangers of its use.

We believe strongly in the paramount importance of educating the public, especially young people and their parents, about the dangers and potentially addictive dynamics of all drugs, including marijuana.

And, while we oppose the use of marijuana as a "medicine" unless it has been approved by the U.S. Food and Drug Administration (FDA), we understand the cannabis plant has some medicinal qualities and support further research.

While there are a number of additional issues and proposals surrounding the wider marijuana debate, we believe our expertise, experience and energy is best applied to educating the public about the dangers of expanded drug and alcohol use as well as the promise and possibility of recovery.

This statement reflects the Hazelden Betty Ford Foundation's clear and singular aim of reducing the harmful impact of addiction.

Reprinted with permission.

The Hazelden Betty Ford Foundation, the largest non-profit provider of prevention, treatment and recover services in the U.S.

Drug Free Australia's Position on Medical Marijuana / Cannabis, July 2014

1. What is the stance of Drug Free Australia on the legalisation of cannabis for medical purposes?

Drug Free Australia (DFA) opposes the legalisation of cannabis for medical purposes because:

- **Its origins have not come from the medical profession, but rather special interest groups and marijuana companies, that can be likened to 'Big Tobacco', where profit is the main motive.**

Groups like the *National Organisation for the Reform of Marijuana Laws* (NORML) have been agitating for medical marijuana for a long time, as has the *Drug Policy Alliance*. However, particular individuals have also put in considerable funds. These include billionaire financier

George Soros and insurance magnate Peter Lewis. It is estimated that Lewis alone has spent between $40 and $60 million on medical marijuana initiatives since the early 80s.[i]

Soros-watcher Rachel Ehrenfeld has described the Soros strategy as set forth to pro- legalisation group *Drug Policy Foundation* in the early nineties:

... in 1993 Soros gave DPF a "set of suggestions to follow if they wanted his assistance: Come up with an approach that emphasizes `treatment and humanitarian endeavors,' he said ... target a few winnable issues, like medical marijuana and the repeal of mandatory minimums." Apparently, they took his advice.[ii]

According to Dr Kevin Sabet, University of Florida: *'Special-interest "Big Tobacco"—like groups and businesses have ensured that marijuana is widely promoted, advertised and commercialized in Colorado. As a result, calls to poison centers have skyrocketed, incidents involving kids going to school with marijuana candy and vaporizers seem more common, and explosions involving butane hash oil extraction have risen. Employers are reporting more workplace incidents involving marijuana use, and deaths have been attributed to ingesting marijuana cookies and food items. Marijuana companies, like their predecessors in the tobacco industry, are determined to keep lining their pockets'.*[iii]

- **Promoters of 'Medical' Marijuana are using the community's compassion for the suffering of sick people; it is emotional blackmail, based on political and economic motives rather than science.**

DFA believes that the current trend in this debate in Australia is mirroring a similar campaign carried out some years ago in the United States, when Dr Robert DuPont spoke against medical marijuana and is quoted as saying:

'More people need to see "medical marijuana" for what it is: a cynical fraud and a cruel hoax. The conflict being discussed at this hearing today, in my view, is not about medicine; it is about the political exploitation of the public's compassion for suffering sick people. Legitimizing smoked marijuana as a "medicine" is a serious threat to the health and safety of all Americans'.[iv]

This is supported by Dr Greg Pike, Adelaide Centre for Bioethics and Culture:
'A dangerous precedent is set by approval processes that are effectively achieved by popular vote of citizens who are not expert judges of medical efficacy, side-effects, abuse potential, or ethics of the doctor-patient relationship. Popular vote is also risky because the public is then at the mercy of pressure from groups who are using medical marijuana as a beachhead for generalised legal access to marijuana'.[v]

- **There are important differences between modern scientific medicine that is administered as single chemicals (usually synthetic) by the oral route of administration and smoked herbal marijuana.**

For example, the Food and Drug Administration, in the United States (similar to the Australian Therapeutic Goods Administration) states that: 'To be accepted as a medicine, the following criteria must be met:

(1) The drug's chemistry must be known and reproducible
(2) There must be adequate safety studies
(3) There must be adequate and well-controlled studies proving efficacy
(4) The drug must be accepted by qualified experts
(5) The scientific evidence must be widely available'.

Cannabis does not meet these criteria.

Other peak organisations such as the *Australian Medical Association*, the *American Medical, Association*, the *American College of Physicians*, the *American Nurses Association*, the *American Cancer Society*, the *American Glaucoma Foundation*, the *National Multiple Sclerosis Society*, the *American Academy of Pediatrics* and the *American Society of Addiction Medicine* all support the approval process and have expressed either opposition to or concern over the use of smoked marijuana as a therapeutic product.

It is important that peak bodies like the FDA in the US and the *Therapeutic Goods Administration* (TGA) in Australia are able to maintain their position as the gatekeepers of the regulatory process by which new medicines become available to the public. They are undermined when, by alternate regulatory means, medicines are made available. This is the case in the US where States have enacted legislation that makes smoked marijuana available for medical purposes without FDA approval'. [vi]

- **There are medications already approved and available to help people who are in pain and suffering that work extremely well**. (Refer to Question 3)
- **Robust research on the harms of cannabis**.

'The scientific verdict is that marijuana can be addictive and dangerous. Despite denials by special interest groups and marijuana businesses, the drug's addictiveness is not debatable: 1 in 6 kids who ever try marijuana will become addicted to the drug, according to the National Institutes of Health. Many baby boomers have a hard time understanding this simply because today's marijuana can be so much stronger than the marijuana of the past.

In fact, more than 450,000 incidents of emergency room admissions related to marijuana occur every year, and heavy marijuana use in adolescence is connected to an 8-point reduction of IQ later in life, irrespective of alcohol use.

Marijuana users also have a six times higher risk of schizophrenia and are significantly more likely to development other psychotic illnesses. It is no wonder that health groups such as the National Alliance of Mental Illness are increasingly concerned about marijuana use and legalization'.[vii]

- **Lack of credible research, especially on smoked marijuana.**

For example: Following the establishment of the *Center for Medicinal Cannabis Research* (CMCR) at the *University of California* in 1999, the number of research projects on smoked cannabis has increased. Several clinical studies have been published on neuropathic pain and experimentally induced pain. In general the results show a modest analgesic effect of smoked cannabis over placebo. It is important to note that most of the subjects in these studies were cannabis experienced, so the results may not be able to be extrapolated to cannabis naïve patients. Moreover, because the subjects were cannabis-experienced, it is likely that blinding was compromised and hence the findings should be interpreted with this in mind.

- **Abuse of the systems in place, where Medical Cannabis has been legalised:**

There seems little doubt that marijuana is being diverted from medical programs for 'recreational' purposes. The *Las Vegas Metropolitan Police Department* recorded an enormous 1200 percent increase in grow site seizures between 2006 and 2010.[viii]

In Colorado, 48.8 percent of adolescents admitted to substance abuse treatment obtained their marijuana from someone registered to use medically.[ix] The authors conclude: Diversion of medical marijuana is common among adolescents in substance treatment. These data support a relationship between medical marijuana exposure and marijuana availability, social norms, frequency of use, substance-related problems and general problems among teens in substance treatment.

In a recent study by Cerda and co-workers, it was found that states with medical marijuana laws had higher rates of use, abuse and dependence.

2. Would DFA consider it for any indications e.g. for people who are terminally ill and in intractable pain and for whom conventional medicines have not worked? Or any other patients with distressing symptoms

DFA would not consider cannabis for any indications for the following reasons: As in Australia, there are no sound scientific studies supported the medical use of marijuana for treatment in the United States and no animal or human data supported the safety or efficacy of marijuana for general medical use.

To quote Dr Stuart Reece, Fellow of Drug Free Australia: '*Approved narcotics work very well in these indications, where many combinations are used in palliative care which are very effective in pain relief. To gain therapeutic effects using cannabis high cannabinoid levels need to be achieved, at which the psychotropic / hallucinogenic effects of cannabis become predominant and are not tolerated by patients who are not used to these effects of cannabis*'.

In the United States, the Food and Drug Administration also concurs that there are alternative (FDA)-approved medications in existence for treatment of many of the proposed uses of smoked marijuana.

3. If not, what alternatives does DFA support?

Currently there are 4 formulations of active ingredients, dronabinol (Marinol), nabilone, nabiximols (Sativex) and rimonabant. The first two are THC lookalikes, whereas Nabiximols is a marijuana extract containing both THC and CBD. Rimonabant is a cannabinoid receptor blocker which was initially marketed as an anti-obesity drug in Europe in 2006 before being withdrawn soon after when side effects including serious depression and suicidal ideation were found to be frequent.

Dronabinol was approved by the US *Food and Drug Administration* (FDA) in 1985 for treating chemotherapy-induced nausea and vomiting and AIDS-related wasting, and although proven effective, both dronabinol and nabilone have not become the mainstays of treatment mainly because of their side effects, which include sedation, anxiety, dizziness, euphoria/dysphoria and hypotension, as well as the presence of superior alternatives.

Dronabinol and nabilone have also been shown to produce symptomatic relief of neuropathic pain and the spasticity associated with multiple sclerosis. However, whilst patients report alleviation of spasticity, measures of objective changes are mixed. In a recent study by Kraft and co-workers, an orally administered extract of cannabis containing mainly THC was found to have no beneficial impact on acute pain and may possibly have enhanced pain sensation. This study highlights not only the complex nature of pain itself, but also the importance of identifying specific therapeutic contexts in which THC may or may not be useful.

It should be noted that while these studies are conducted much like other studies on medical agents, a particular problem arises because the psychoactive side effects of dronabinol and nabilone make it difficult to maintain appropriate blinding, which is a basic requirement of a randomized controlled trial. In other words, when the research subjects become aware that they are receiving the active ingredient and not the placebo, their perception of therapeutic value is potentially confounded and a study's claim of therapeutic advantage over placebo may be compromised.

Nabiximols is an interesting example of a novel form of delivery by nasal spray that has the advantage of rapid absorption. By including both THC and CBD together, it may be that CBD limits some of the adverse side effects common with THC alone. It has been licensed for the treatment of cancer pain and neuropathic pain.

The role of CBD in potentially mitigating some of the adverse effects of THC may prove to be a valuable finding. It also highlights why use of the raw herbal product could be even more problematic than already thought, because as new strains have been developed, the amount of THC has risen at the same time as the amount of CBD has declined. In some strains, CBD is virtually absent. When production of cannabis is permitted by the public for medical use, there is no control over the levels of active ingredients and in particular the ratio of THC to CBD.

One final variation on delivery systems involves vaporization of the herbal product. This means of delivery is about as close as possible to smoked marijuana. Some clinical trials are currently underway.

It is important to note that with each of these formulations little is known about the medium to long term adverse effects. However, given that there is evidence for long-term harm arising from studies of those who smoke cannabis regularly, significant caution should be exercised about these formulations of active ingredients'.[xi]

DFA supports the use of approved alternatives such as Nabiximols (also known as Sativex). If they need to be made more accessible and less costly, Australia has a PBS process that could be employed to assist.

4. Do you think there is a place for medical cannabis if it is strictly controlled e.g prescribed by doctors and dispensed by pharmacists?

DFA's findings from examples in the United States where cannabis has been legalised show that strict controls are not working. For example:

- Increased use of marijuana
- Laws abused
- Taxation benefits lower than expected

5. Is DFA comfortable with the use of the drugs morphine, amphetamine, ketamine and cocaine for medical purposes, as allowed now in Australia?

When used for medical purposes, having been authorised by the TGA, these drugs are acceptable. Cannabis however, is far more complex and components far more difficult to control. For example, while opium has been recognised for its medicinal value for many centuries, the active ingredients codeine and morphine have now been extracted and subjected to extensive research and analysis over many years. We now have both in various formulations with known dosage and purity, a body of information on side-effects, known indications and contraindications, knowledge of therapeutic targets, patient populations for whom treatment is appropriate, and knowledge of abuse potential. No medical authority would ever prescribe or even recommend smoking opium, not only because of the availability of formulations of active ingredients which are superior, but also because of the harm of smoking as a delivery system.[xii]

6. If not, what alternatives does DFA support?
The use of approved drugs as described in Questions 2 and 3.

7. Would DFA support a trial into the use of medical cannabis in Australia?
DFA would not support a trial for the following reasons:

- All of the above. Plus:
- The system that is in place through the Therapeutic Goods Administration should not be bypassed. We have enough ethically and legally authorised pharmaceutical medicines that assist medical responses to pain and suffering available
- As stated in question 1, there is an abundance of research, information and emerging trends with negative outcomes from locations where medical cannabis has been introduced, especially in the United States. Regarding the direct health effects of cannabis, Nora Volkow MD, NIDA, has produced 'Adverse Health Effects of Marijuana Use' gives current data that has been well researched.[xiii]

This is more than sufficient for Australia to use as a gauge, without having to introduce trials here.

....

References

i O'Connor C, High Roller: How Billionaire Peter Lewis Is Bankrolling Marijuana Legalization, Forbes Magazine, April 2012 See *http://www.forbes.com/sites/clareoconnor*

ii Rachel Ehrenfeld, May 1996, The Movement to Legalize Drugs in the United States: Who's Behind It? Downloaded from the Capital Research website *www.capitalresearch.com*

iii *http://edition.cnn.com/2014/07/10/opinion/sabet-colorado-marijuana/*

iv *http://www.ibhinc.org/pdfs/RLDMedMJTestimony031407.pdf*

v Pike G, Medical Marijuana, *May, 2013*

vi Pike Op Cit 2013

vii Kevin Sabet http://edition.cnn.com/2014/07/10/opinion/sabet-colorado-marijuana

viii Raybuck T, Medical Marijuana, Nevada's Big Gamble. *The Journal of Global Drug Policy and Practice* 5(2), 2011

ix Thurstone C, Lieberman SA & Schmiege SJ, Medical marijuana diversion and associated problems in adolescent substance treatment. *Drug Alcohol Dependence* 118(2-3):489-492, 2011

x Cerda M *et al.*, Medical marijuana laws in 50 states: investigating the relationship between state legalization of medical marijuana and marijuana use, abuse and dependence, *Drug Alcohol Depend.* 120(1-3): 22-27, 2012

xi Pike, Op. Cit 2013

xii Pike, Op Cit 2013

xiii Nora D. Volkow, M.D., Ruben D. Baler, Ph.D., Wilson M. Compton, M.D., and Susan R.B. Weiss, Ph.D.

Adverse Health Effects of Marijuana Use', N Engl J Med 2014; 370:2219-2227June 5, 2014. For more information go to www.drugfree.org.au

Provided by Jo Baxter, Drug Free Australia.

EDWARD GOGEK, MD
Arizona, USA

Legalization Always Increases Use

Shortly after the 2012 election, when Colorado and Washington voted to legalize marijuana, *Atlantic* magazine interviewed pro-marijuana campaign managers to hear how they had won. They had done it by focusing on women, especially moms. Their advertising campaign promised four benefits: "Fewer profits for drug cartels. Increased funding for schools. More time for police to 'focus on violent crime.'" And "their children would not be affected."[1]

Parents do not want their kids using marijuana. So the marijuana lobby had to convince moms that legalization would make it harder for kids to get the drug.

A RAND Corporation report that studied California's 2010 legalization initiative concluded that, if it passed, prices would go down, and availability and consumption would both go up by 50–100 percent.[2] Other research has shown that when young people live in areas with higher concentrations of alcohol outlets, they're more likely to drink, even though it's illegal for them to do so. And when the drinking age is lowered to 18, it results in 16 and 17-year-olds drinking a lot more.[3] For any drug, increased access equals increased use.

The marijuana lobby has to convince voters that the normal law of supply and demand doesn't apply, and that the way to keep teenagers from using marijuana is to legalize it. So they came up with the idea that we should regulate it like alcohol. In Colorado, they even named the proposed amendment to the state constitution, *The Regulate Marijuana Like Alcohol Act of 2012*,[4] and ran ads reading: "Please, card my son. Regulate the sale of marijuana and help me keep it out of his hands."[5]

When the *Monitoring the Future* study asked 8th, 10th, and 12th grade students which drugs were easy to obtain, at every grade level more students said alcohol and tobacco were easy to get.[6] Legal drugs are always more readily available than illegal ones. Why? Because legal drugs are available at every corner market and in most homes.

However, there's something wrong with this whole comparison. If we want to know how hard it is for teenagers to buy illegal drugs, we shouldn't be using marijuana as our example. In Canada and the United States, marijuana is practically legal.

If we want to see whether keeping a drug illegal makes it harder for teenagers to buy, we have to look at drugs that are prescription only or truly illegal. Students at all grade levels say alcohol and marijuana are relatively easy to obtain while prescription drugs and truly illegal drugs are much harder to get. And the difference is significant. Among high school seniors, about 20 percent say cocaine, meth, and heroin are easy to find. For alcohol and marijuana, it's more than 80 percent.

Despite what the marijuana lobby told voters in Colorado and Washington, legal drugs are always more widely used. History bears this out:

In 2011 and 2012, the Florida legislature, along with several Florida cities and counties, banned the sale of synthetic drugs such as bath salts. Within a year, Florida emergency rooms reported a significant drop in the number of people coming in for treatment because of these drugs.[7]

Prohibition of alcohol is routinely labeled a failure, but when the United States made alcohol illegal in the 1920s, use dropped by two-thirds. It increased again over time, but even at the end of Prohibition, alcohol use was still much lower than it had been before the law was introduced.[8] And it wasn't just social drinking that declined, hardcore alcoholism did, too. Deaths from cirrhosis dropped by nearly two-thirds, and drunk and disorderly arrests were cut in half.[9] In the ten years after the act's repeal, alcohol use in the United States doubled.

One of the grimmest experiments in drug legalization occurred in 1858, when the British defeated China in the Second Opium War and forced the Chinese to legalize the drug. Their aim was to fund their other colonial adventures by selling opium to the Chinese people and, sadly, it was a great success.[10] Kathleen Lodwick,[11] a Penn State history professor who has written a book about the opium trade in China, said that after legalization "use of the drug skyrocketed." Millions became addicted. At one point, 27 percent of China's adult male population used opium regularly.[12]

Shortly after the state of Washington allowed the sale of recreational marijuana, local public radio station NWPR interviewed one buyer who said he hadn't used marijuana in twenty years, but was using it again because it was legal.[13]

However, the best evidence that legalizing marijuana increases teenage use comes from the U.S. states that legalized medical marijuana. Research shows that marijuana use is higher in states with these laws, but more significantly, teenage marijuana use is increasing faster in these states. Over six years, teenage use in medical marijuana states went up by 30 percent. In states without these laws, it only increased 5 percent.

There is no way to make marijuana legal for adults without also making it easily available to teenagers. That's what the research tells us, and it's what our experience with alcohol and tobacco should make obvious.

....

Endnotes

1 http://www.theatlantic.com/politics/archive/2012/11/the-secret-ingredients-for-marijuana-legalization-moms-and-hispanics/265369/

2 http://www.rand.org/pubs/testimonies/CT351.html

3 Huckle, T.; Huakau, J.; Sweetsur, P.; et al. Density of alcohol outlets and teenage drinking: Living in an alcogenic environment is associated with

higher consumption in a metropolitan setting. Addiction 103:1614–1621, 2008. PMID: 18821871

Huckle, T.; You, R.Q.; and Casswell, S. Increases in quantities consumed in drinking occasions in New Zealand 1995–2004. Drug and Alcohol Review 30:366–371, 2010. PMID: 21355906

4 http://www.regulatemarijuana.org/s/regulate-marijuana-alcohol-act-2012

5 http://www.regulatemarijuana.org/regulation-works

6 http://www.monitoringthefuture.org//pubs/monographs/mtf-vol1_2012.pdf

7 http://www.drugfree.org/join-together/experts-say-bans-on-synthetic-drugs-in-florida-have-reduced-sales/?utm_source=Join%20Together%20Daily&utm_campaign=0359b39517-JT_Daily_News_Alcoholism_and_PTSD&utm_medium=email&utm_term=0_97f4d27738-0359b39517-221989089

8 http://www.goodreads.com/work/quotes/8912086-last-call-the-rise-and-fall-of-prohibition

9 http://www.nytimes.com/1989/10/16/opinion/actually-prohibition-was-a-success.html

10 http://www.psu.edu/ur/archives/SOCIETY_POLITICS/Opium.html

11 http://en.wikipedia.org/wiki/Kathleen_L._Lodwick

12 https://muse.jhu.edu/login?auth=0&type=summary&url=/journals/bulletin_of_the_history_of_medicine/v071/71.4br_lodwick.html

13 http://nwpr.org/post/marijuana-scarce-wash-pot-industry 9-9-14

Ed Gogek, MD, received his medical training in both Canada and the United States. He graduated from the University of Illinois, College of Medicine, and followed with a residency in psychiatry at the Maine Medical Center and at the University of Western, Ontario.

In 30 years as a psychiatrist, Dr. Gogek has worked in prisons, homeless clinics, community mental health centers, private practice and in many substance abuse treatment programs. More recently, Dr. Gogek was a board member of KeepAZDrugFree, a committee opposing Arizona's 2010 medical marijuana ballot measure. Dr. Gogek is the author of *Marijuana Debunked* (2015).

LYNETTE CROW-IVERSON

What is the Societal Impact of Legalized Marijuana?

In Colorado, we are asking ourselves, "Now that recreational marijuana is legal … how do we prepare ourselves for the social outcomes that are not a part of the marijuana marketing scheme?"

The answer to this question is far from simple. Because we are the first state to legalize recreational marijuana use, we have enrolled ourselves into front-running the experience of having to become keenly aware of the various social outcomes that the legalization of recreational marijuana could imply. As we continue to learn through the experiences and outcomes of this legislation in our state, our goal is to be a model. Models present lessons learned that become best practices.

So, what are some of the best practices other states will benefit from in watching Colorado's efforts? Below are items that we in Colorado are either already facing—or will be facing in the days ahead. This is food for thought, for those considering the same question:

What does substance abuse cost employers?
According to the Substance Abuse and Mental Health Services Administration (SAMHSA):

- Substance abusers are 2.5x more likely to be absent from work 8 or more days a year
- Substance abusers are 1/3 less productive on the job
- Substance abuse costs employers $7,000/month annually in lost revenue
- Approximately 40% of all Worker's Compensation claims are related to substance abuse
- 80% of drug abusers self-report that they steal from their workplaces to support their habit
- 90% of current, full-time workers with alcohol or illicit drug dependence work for small businesses that are less likely to enforce employee screening policies
- Drug use costs U.S. businesses upwards of $100 billion annually

In a 2010 study by the National Drug Free Workplace Alliance, employees testing positive for marijuana had an absentee rate of 75% higher than those whose test results were negative (National Drug-Free Workplace Alliance).

According to U.S. Dept. of Health and Human Services, employees who test positive for marijuana use have 55%

more industrial accidents and 85% more injuries (Burlington).

It is clear that estimating healthcare-related costs directly resulting from marijuana use can and will be staggering in the years ahead. Mechanisms are not yet in place to specifically track this data due to the lack of funding strategies and/or responsible agencies that could potentially serve as a clearinghouse for maintaining appropriate documentation.

Colorado's Amendment 64 states, "Nothing in this section is intended to require an employer to permit or accommodate the use, consumption, possession, transfer, display, transportation, sale or growing of marijuana in the workplace or to affect the ability of employers to have policies **restricting** the use of marijuana by employees (Vicente)."

Essentially, this protects the employer's right to enforce their drug policies; however, marijuana industry representatives have made proposals to overturn employer's rights through legal efforts that will play out in the court system. This will cost employer's untold expenses in defending their safe and drug free workplace policies against those who intend to create new precedents in favor of employee drug use (Ryan). Nonetheless, keeping employers rights intact has proven to be a best practice in protecting Colorado businesses from the consequences of on-the-job marijuana use and influence.

Social costs to the community

Tobacco is legal and regulated. Its use is also our nation's No. 1 cause of preventable death. Tobacco use costs our country at least $200 billion annually—which is about 10 times the amount of money our state and federal governments collect from today's taxes on cigarettes and other tobacco products (CDC).

Alcohol is legal and regulated. Its use is our nation's No. 3 cause of preventable death, behind diet-related illness. Alcohol use costs our country at least $185 billion annually —which is also roughly 10 times the amount of money our state and federal governments collect from today's taxes on the substance (HHS).

Marijuana: According to the 2010 National Study on Drug Use and Health (NSDUH):

- Marijuana accounted for 4.5 million of the estimated 7.1 million Americans dependent on or abusing illicit drugs
- In 2009, approximately 18 percent of people aged 12 and older entering drug abuse treatment programs reported marijuana as their primary drug of abuse
- 61 percent of persons under 15 reported marijuana as their primary drug of abuse

We cannot currently estimate the costs of legal recreational marijuana when it comes to prevention, addiction, treatment and recovery: best practices are not yet known, and there are no medications that have been proven to help with treatment. We will have many years ahead of us, and countless accounts of trial and error, before we know what works; and we will spend millions of dollars before we figure it out.

In fiscal year 2012, the State of Colorado collected $5.4 million in sales tax on "medical marijuana" purchases. This sounds great—until you consider that Colorado also experienced a $5.7 million budget shortfall because of medical marijuana regulation (Gallagher). The budget shortfall meant a great deal of regulation simply didn't happen. Though Colorado policymakers agreed 55 full-time state employees would be sufficient to regulate medical marijuana, the state received revenues to employ only 15 full-time employees.

Barbara Brohl, executive director of the Colorado Department of Revenue, stated, "The funding model just didn't work. And, as a result, the division wasn't able to perform the regulatory and oversight functions it was created to do."

A growing trend that OBGYN providers are seeing is wide-spread marijuana use amongst pregnant women to treat nausea. Studies show that cannabis easily crosses the placental barrier to the fetus. Babies can test positive for marijuana up to 3 weeks after birth. Cannabis is excreted in breast milk, and can interfere with fetal brain development. For children who were exposed to marijuana in utero, we see hyperactivity disorder at 10 years of age (Jaques). At 12 years of age, children who were exposed in utero struggle with higher cognitive processes and suffer early onset depression and mental illness (Goldschmidt). These issues will contribute to further social costs for treatment and special education needs.

Another social cost we face is the increased number of applications for public assistance. It is not simply the individual who tests positive for marijuana and is fired, Colorado has seen a significant spike in out-of-state transfers who cannot find work. In other words, Colorado is attracting those who move to the state in order to use recreational marijuana legally; however, without being able to secure jobs, the Colorado Department of Human Services has been deluged with requests for public assistance that one employee called "a crushing load". Food banks are preparing for a burden like they have never seen in the state's history.

Additionally, local law enforcement agencies are strapped for funding to provide road side sobriety testing that includes blood draws for marijuana impairment. Consider that drivers have a two-fold risk of crashes while driving marijuana impaired. In a recent national Healthy Kids survey, 11% of kids say they have driven impaired in the last week (NIDA). In both Colorado and Washington, law enforcement agencies report that marijuana impairment is on the rise; however, they do not have the resources to test or track numbers – therefore the data is incomplete as to the social impact, direct burden and related costs.

Yet another item of concern is the regulatory costs pertaining to safe products. Whether this refers to grow operations, edibles, safety packaging or promoting products to adolescents, marijuana is not currently subject to the same standards as tobacco or alcohol and is without any oversight jurisdiction. The Food and Drug Administration is not responsible for safe marijuana products at the federal level, so what are the states to do? In Colorado it is the Department of Revenue that has oversight of recreational marijuana. What does the Department of Revenue know about such issues as inspection for molds, pesticides, herbicides and additives or child-proof packaging laws? Since there is not a plan for recreational marijuana to generate funding for these issues, it is incumbent upon the state budget office to create solutions from the General Fund, effectively taking needed monies from schools, road improvement projects, parks, public safety, etc. Again, it will take years to understand the social and fiscal impact to the state.

Direct healthcare costs

We must consider the long-term outcomes of healthcare associated costs with increased marijuana consumption. In a 2014 public health symposium sponsored by Denver Public Health, a few highlights included the following concerns (these are not comprehensive):

- Marijuana Users & Cancer Risks (Bowles) (Mehra) (Callaghan) (Marks)
- Smoke contains hundreds of combustion products that increase risk of cancer among users
- Marijuana users are at risk for increased lung cancer
- Increased oral and tongue cancer risks persists for those who smoke marijuana
- Marijuana Use & Heart Disease, Stroke & Lung Disease (Mittleman) (Frost) (Wolff) (Barber)
- Acute increases in heart rate and blood pressure; myocardial infarction risk within first hour after use
- Cerebral narrowing increases risk of stroke
- 2x risk of bronchial disease and chronic obstructive pulmonary disease (COPD), lung cancer

- Decreased lung function
- Marijuana Use & Mental Health (Burns) (Meier, Persistent cannabis users show neuropsychological decline from childhood to midlife) (Lev-Ran) (Moore) (Hayatbakhsh) (VanLaar)
- Early onset of schizophrenia for adolescents – 2-3x higher
- Shortened time to psychosis and psychotic episodes – 40% higher (all users)
- Structural brain changes to hippocampus long-term (adult and adolescent)
- Neuropsychological decline, cognitive decline (adolescents), IQ loss
- 17% increased risk for depression—all users
- Increased anxiety and depression for all users
- Unintentional Exposure in Children (Want) (Wang)
- Marijuana poisonings amongst children has spiked for ER visits to Children's Hospital Colorado.
- 1-3 children/month since 2009—total 985 exposures
- Symptoms show up 2–24 hours after exposures and last from hours to 4 days
- Edibles are greatest risk factor. Colorado set the lowest standards for packaging possible by law
- Only states with legalized medical marijuana have had child exposures

Future costs

Studies show that when young people perceive less risk involved in an activity, their participation in that activity increases. According to the Monitoring the Future Survey of 2013, 60% of high school seniors say that marijuana is not harmful. Directly related to social messaging that marijuana is "safe", ⅓ of high school seniors report smoking marijuana in the past year and 6.5% of high school seniors report they smoke marijuana daily. For the first time, marijuana use is higher than tobacco use amongst teens in the U.S (Johnston).

MRI scans of the corpus callosum, the bundle of fibers that connects the two brain hemispheres and allows the two hemispheres to communicate and work in a coordinated way, have been compared among young adult males who smoked marijuana daily (and started at an average age of 15 yrs) along with age-matched non-users (Arnone). The scan of the daily user shows thinner corpus callosum fibers than the scan of the non-user indicating that there are white matter integrity issues for the daily user. This means structural changes to the brain. These changes in the brain structure (especially the hippocampus) of people exposed to marijuana during adolescence are significant to long-term success. For example, poorer communication across different parts of the brain that need to work together for proper cognition may cause cognitive disorders such as schizophrenia.

Ultimately, what does this mean? Persistent, dependent use before age 18 causes lasting harm to intelligence, attention and memory.

Adolescents who use marijuana before the age of 18 are 2-4 times more likely to develop symptoms of psychosis in early adulthood than those who do not. This finding has been replicated at least eight times and persists after controlling for many possible confounding variables such as family history, other substance use, and socioeconomic status. These studies have involved thousands and thousands of people over generations and in several populations and countries.

Longitudinal studies in Amsterdam have shown that chronic adolescent use of marijuana may result in as much as 8 points of IQ loss that are not re-gained throughout the individual's lifetime. While 8 IQ points may not sound like a lot ... on a scale where 100 is the mean, a loss from an IQ of 100 to 92 represents a drop from being in the 50th percentile to being in the 29th. Higher IQ correlates with higher education and income, better health, and a longer life. Someone who loses 8 IQ points as an adolescent may be disadvantaged compared to their same-age peers for years to come (Meier, Persistent cannabis users show neropsychological decline from childhood to midlife).

Consider these findings for the impact of marijuana on adolescent users:

- Early onset of schizophrenia for adolescents is 2-3x higher
- Shortened time to psychosis and psychotic episodes is 40% higher
- Neuropsychological decline and cognitive decline that cannot be recovered

- 17% increased risk for depression and anxiety
- Less school achievement and increased high school dropout rates
- Increased risky sexual behaviors, such as not using a condom
- Psychologically and physically addictive with 1 in 6 adolescents developing marijuana dependence syndrome
- Aggression and withdrawal that frequently includes restlessness, nervousness, agitation and insomnia
- Accidents are the leading cause of death for adolescents, and marijuana use predicts an increased risk of accidents by 30%, particularly when driving
- Marijuana has acute, sub-acute, and long-term effects on cognition and memory

We have not seen the full consequences of the legalization of recreational marijuana. Yet, knowing what we do about the social and financial costs and outcomes that we now face and will begin to face in the near future, what steps can we take to prepare ourselves?

We can all continue to support prevention efforts to protect and educate our youth; we can all fight to protect employers' rights to enforce drug policies; and we can all exercise our rights as citizens to stay informed on the impacts of legalized marijuana on our state and vote for a safer future.

Bilbiography

Arnone, Barrick, Chengappa. "Corpus callosum damage in heavy marijuana use: Preliminary evidence from diffusion tensor tractography and tract-based spatial statistics." *NeuroImage* (2008): 41:1067-1074.

Barber. "Cannabis, ischemic stroke and transient ischemic attack: a case-control study." *Stroke* (2013): 44:2327-2329.

Bowles. "The intersection between cannabis and cancer in the U.S." *Critical Review in Oncology and Hematology* (2012): 83:1-10.

Burlington, D. Bruce. *Testimony on Federal Workplace Drug-Testing.* Washington D.C.: DHHS, 1998.

Burns, J. "Pathway from cannabis to psychosis: A review of evidence." *Frontiers in Psychiatry* (2013): 4:128-1-12.

Callaghan. "Marijuana use and risk of lung cancer: a 40 years cohort study." *Cancer Causes and Control* (2013): 24:1811-1820.

CDC. *Centers for Disease Control.* 2007. 4 April 2014. <www.cdc.gov/tobacco/data_statistics/fact_sheet>.

Frost. "Marijuana and long-term mortality among survivors of acute myocardial infarction." *American Heart Journal* (2013): 165:170-175.

Gallagher, Dennis. *Medical Marijuana Licensing.* Denver: Office of the City Auditor, 2013.

Goldschmidt. "Effects of prenatal marijuana exposure on child behavior problems at age 10." *Neurotoxicol* (2000): 325-336.

Hayatbakhsh, M. "Cannabis and anxiety and depression in young adults: A large prospective study." *American Academy Child Adolescent Psychiatry* (2007): 408-417.

HHS. *The Economic Costs of Alcohol Abuse.* Washington D.C.: National Institute of Health, 2000.

Jaques, S. "Cannabis, the pregnant woman and her child: weeding out the myths." *Perinatology* (2014): 1-8.

Johnston, L. *Key Findings on Adolescent Drug Use.* Ann Arbor: NIDA, 2013.

Lev-Ran, S. "The association between cannabis use and depression: a systematic review and meta-analysis of longitudinal studies." *Psychological Medicine* (2014): 44:797-810.

Marks. "Association of marijuana smoking with oropharyngeal and oral tongue cancers." *Cancer Epidemiology, Biomarkers and Prevention* (2013): 23:160-171.

Mehra. "The association between marijuana smoking and lung cancer." *Archives of Internal Medicine* (2006): 166:1359-67.

Meier, M. "Persistent cannabis users show neropsychological decline from childhood to midlife." *PNAS* (2012): e2657-64.

———. "Persistent cannabis users show neuropsychological decline from childhood to midlife." *PNAS* (2012): e2657-64.

Mittleman. "Triggering myocardial infarction by marijuana." *Circulation* (2001): 103:2805-2809.

Moore, T. "Cannabis use and risk of psychotic or affective mental health outcomes." *Lancet* (2007): 319-328.

National Drug-Free Workplace Alliance. 2010. 4 April 2014. <www.ndwa.org/statistics.php>.

NIDA. *National Institute on Drug Abuse*. 2013. April 2014. <http://www.drugabuse.gov/publications/drugfacts/drugged-driving>.

NSDUH. *Center for Behavioral Health Statistics and Quality*. 2010. 4 April 2014. <https://nsduhweb.rti.org/respweb>.

Ryan, Kimberlie. *Minority Report, Implementation of Amendment 64, Exhibit A*. Denver: CO Governor's Office Task Force, 2013.

SAMHSA. *Substance Abuse and Mental Health Safety Administration*. 2005. 4 April 2014. <http://www.samhsa.gov/data/trends/htm>.

VanLaar, M. "Does cannabis use predict the first incidence of mood and anxiety disorders in the adult population?" *Addiction* (2007): 1251-1260.

Vicente, et.al. *Amendment 64, Article XVIII of the Constitution of the state of Colorado*. Denver, 2012.

Wang, GS. "Association of unintentional pediatric exposures with decriminlization of marijuana in the U.S." *Annals of Emergency Medicine* (2014): 63:1450-55.

Want, GS. "Pediatric marijuana exposures in a medical marijuana state." *JAMA Pediatrics* (2013): 167:630-633.

Wolff. "Cannabis-related stroke. Myth or Reality?" *Stroke* (2013): 44:558-563.

Lynette Crow-Iverson is an innovator in the field of pre-employment screening and substance abuse prevention; promoting hiring excellence in today's workforce. The owner and creator of Conspire! Ms. Crow was appointed as a committee member for the Colorado Springs Chamber of Commerce Healthcare Council to evaluate the healthcare system both locally and nationally. Lynette is currently serving as a trustee for the Colorado Springs Healthcare Foundation Board, and The Pikes Peak Work Force Board.

DR. ANDRA SMITH, PH.D
Associate Professor, School of Psychology, University of Ottawa

An Example of Marijuana's Impact on Teen Brain Activity

'I LOVE DRIVING man but wow it is hard to stop when I know that yellow light has been yellow for a while and will be red as I get to the stop line. And forget about remembering where I parked my car at the gym when I come out.'

This quote, spoken by a participant in a functional MRI (fMRI) research study, highlights two important types of cognition that are impacted by regular use of marijuana by teens. Participant X was a member of the Ottawa Prenatal Prospective study (OPPS) and had been smoking marijuana on a regular basis (>3 days/week) since the age of 13. He was 19 at the time and was about to have his brain scanned while performing 4 cognitive tasks. Two of the tasks would test his ability to inhibit responding and his visuospatial working memory. The other two tasks would measure his verbal working memory and cognitive interference.

The OPPS

The OPPS is a longitudinal study that was initially designed to investigate the impact of prenatal drug exposures, particularly marijuana, on the offspring of predominantly middle class families (Fried, 1995). A benefit of this type of research is that the children were followed and tested throughout their lives every 2-3 years, providing a priceless database of lifestyle variables, behavioural measures and drug exposure information. This accumulated information included data on the offsprings' own drug use, including when they began using and how much they had used over the years. This invaluable information allowed for an assessment of not only the long term impact of prenatal exposure to marijuana on cognition but also the impact of current use of the sample as young adults.

Neuropsychological test results from the OPPS were obtained at ages 9-12, 13-16 and 17-20 years (Fried et al., 1998; Fried et al., 2003; Fried et al., 2005). This extensive prospective information is unprecedented and includes over 4000 lifestyle variables that can be included or controlled for in statistical analyses. At 17-20 years of age, taking into account premorbid results, heavy marijuana users (>5 joints/week for more than 1 year) showed two strong negative associations in the domains of memory and speed of visual processing (Fried et al., 2005). Although results for other neurocognitive domains were not significant, there were trends and these subtle impacts were the impetus for the fMRI study.

fMRI

fMRI is a neuroimaging technique that provides for a window into the brain as it works. Images of the brain, as it performs cognitive tasks, can shed light on patterns of brain activity, including circuitry and networks that work together during a specific type of processing, such as working memory. It is a non-invasive technique with no injections of radioactive contrast agents and has excellent spatial and temporal resolution. An important advantage of fMRI as a compliment to neuropsychological assessment is that the results can reveal differences in brain activity patterns between groups of participants despite similar performance outcomes. Similar performance (reaction times and errors) does not mean similar brain activity and this sensitivity of fMRI to identify altered neural activity makes it ideal for uncovering the brain regions and neurocircuitry vulnerable to marijuana smoked in adolescents.

Executive Functioning

The cognitive processes impacted in the OPPS sample and those found to be jeopardized in other samples fall under the umbrella term of executive functions. Executive functioning includes several types of neural processes, such as organizing, planning, decision making and providing the higher cognitive thought to perform goal directed behaviours. These are critical for humans to succeed academically, financially, in relationships and in the workplace. The teen years are critical and an ideal time to optimize the development of this type of neurocognitive ability. One reason for this is that the prefrontal cortex is still under construction in these years. This is the part of the brain that really distinguishes humans from other animals and allows for information processing that involves higher order cognition, including imparting rational thoughts onto emotional situations. Along with its intact connections with the rest of the brain, the successful development of the prefrontal cortex is central to the establishment of effective executive functioning. This requires significant strengthening of connections in the brain through myelination (fatty insulation around neurons), increasing the speed of transmission of neural information and ultimately achieving maximal communication between brain regions. This is paralleled by a process called pruning that might seem counterintuitive but that also helps sculpt the cytoarchitecture of the brain to allow for increasing maturity in thought and action. Inefficient connections that are not used are eliminated, making room for the efficient, myelinated neurons. These two critical neurodevelopment stages of the young brain are potentially high jacked by the use of marijuana in adolescents.

Methodology

Thirty-five OPPS young adults (19-21 years of age) completed the fMRI research, however, due to other illicit drug use (as comfirmed by urine analysis and through self-report), or structural anomaly only 24 participants were included in the final results. Although a small sample, results were significant at stringent levels of probability. Participants were all right handed, had English as their first language, and did not meet diagnostic criteria for an Axis I diagnosis from the Diagnostic and Statistical Manual of Mental Disorders (DSM-IV). In addition, all participants met fMRI compatibility criteria, including no claustrophobia, no metal implants, no pacemaker, no recent surgery, and suitable vision for viewing stimuli.

Regular marijuana use was defined as smoking more than 1 marijuana cigarette per week for at least three years. The resulting sample consisted of ten marijuana users (six males, four females, mean age 20) and fourteen non-using controls (nine males, five females, mean age of 20). The users reported smoking an average of 11.48 marijuana joints per week (ranging from 2 – 37.5 joints per week) for an average of 4.55 years. This level of marijuana use would approximate a lifetime average of 2697 joints smoked, which is considered very heavy exposure (Bava et al., 2009). Participants in the nonusers group reported never using marijuana regularly. Although three of the fourteen nonusers reported sporadic use, it was no more than one to four times over the past year. No participants had used illicit drugs on a regular basis or within a month before fMRI testing, which included no use of amphetamines, crack, cocaine, heroin, mushrooms, hashish, lysergic acid, steroids, solvents, and tranquilizers. Seven of the ten marijuana users reported regular use of nicotine, while no participants in the nonusers group reported smoking cigarettes on a regular basis. Therefore, nicotine use was controlled for in all statistical analyses.

The four fMRI tasks were presented to participants on

a screen at the foot of the patient table, which participants viewed through a mirror mounted on the head coil of the 1.5 T Siemens Magnetom Symphony MR. Participants responded to instructions using a 4 button MRI compatible fibre optic-response pad. The tasks included two working memory tasks, one a letter 2-back task and one a visuospatial 2-back task. The other two tasks were challenging neurocircuitry involved in cognitive interference and impulsivity, including a Counting Stroop task and a Go/No Go task, respectively.

Task Descriptions

The n-back working memory task requires neural activity involved in a set of mental processes including the storage and manipulation of information (letters or symbols in multiple parts of the screen for example) for a short amount of time, followed by retrieval. It is a means for facilitating goal-directed higher-order cognitive processes like planning and learning, as well as reasoning and comprehension. All behaviours required for success in society. Neuroimaging studies have confirmed that the 2-back version of the task measures working memory and has been adapted for visuospatial, as well as letter processing.

The letter n-back task for this study included letters presented one at a time on the screen (1 every 2 seconds) with instructions to either press when an X was presented (baseline condition) or press when the same letter that was presented 2 stimuli prior was presented again (test/working memory condition). Subtracting all images of the baseline condition from the working memory condition yields the brain activity related only to working memory. A similar subtraction is performed for the visuospatial version of the task that was used with the OPPS participants in the same fMRI session. A zero was presented on the screen in 9 different positions, one at a time, and the instructions for the baseline condition were to press when the zero was in the middle of the screen while the working memory condition instructions were to press when the zero was presented in the same position it had been seen in 2 stimuli prior.

The other two tasks presented in the scanner were a Go/No Go task that presented letters one at a time on the screen (1/second) with instructions to press for X for baseline and then press for all letters except X for the response inhibition trials. There were 50% Xs presented so a prepotent response was to press for X and when asked to not press for X response inhibition circuitry is more challenged. The Counting Stroop engages a similar response inhibition circuitry but also tests cognitive interference. The task consists of congruent and incongruent blocks. The congruent stimuli were names of common animals (i.e. dog, cat, bird, or mouse), whereas during incongruent trials, the stimulus words were number words (i.e. one, two, three, or four). During each trial, participants were presented with 1 to 4 identical words printed in white on a black background, which presented horizontally one above another. They were instructed to indicate the number of words observed for each group using the appropriate button on the response pad (index finger for one word, middle finger for two words, etc.). Stimulus words were common words from each of the two semantic categories and were balanced for word length. For example, if dog was presented on 3 lines on the screen (congruent) the participant pressed with their ring finger, similarly, the same response would be required if the word two was presented on 3 lines also (incongruent). Accessing the cognitive interference neural networks was accomplished by subtracting the neural activity for the incongruent minus the congruent trials.

These two tasks involve processing required for withholding responding when inappropriate, being able to block out interfering stimulation and controlling impulsive behaviour. These behaviours underlie so many aspects of socially acceptable behaviour that impairment can lead to problems with relationships, the law, school and employment.

Consistent Imaging Results

Although each of the 4 tasks assessed different types of processing, they all fall under the category of executive functioning. Interestingly, each task indicated that regular use of marijuana was related to increased activity in widespread brain regions, including the prefrontal cortex, while no performance deficits were observed. fMRI tasks are designed to ensure participants are able to perform them and thus the resulting brain activity differences, despite performance similarities, can be interpreted as a quantifiable measure of significant neurophysiological impact of marijuana use on executive functioning. More specifically, during response inhibition (Go/No Go task), more activity was related to more marijuana exposure in the thalamus, premotor cortex, dorsolateral prefrontal cortex, precuneus and inferior parietal lobule (Smith et al., 2011). These areas contribute to response inhibition but also include other areas not typically associated with this type of processing. The increased activity and recruitment of other areas suggests a form of compensation required to perform the task successfully. This was similar for the Counting Stroop whereby increased activity was observed in typical interference related brain regions, like the cingulate gyrus, but then also in areas not typically associated with this type of task, such as the rolandic operculum (Hatchard et al., in press). Both working memory tasks revealed augmented blood flow in the dorsolateral prefrontal cortex and several temporal lobe regions (Smith et al., 2010).

Interpretation of Results

This compensation, with increased activity and recruitment of other regions, to perform the tasks, despite no performance differences, demonstrates the benefit of using fMRI to understand the impact of marijuana on the brain. This information also provides valuable insight into the extra demands placed on the brain of a marijuana user, particularly a young user. If marijuana impacts the development of imperative neurophysiological processes, like neuronal pruning of unnecessary connections and myelination of dorsolateral prefrontal cortex neurons, this would impact negatively the executive control the brain has on behaviour. By increasing blood flow to the necessary areas the brain could work harder to perform tasks to success. However, when these neural systems are challenged or more demands are put on them during more real life situations, the brain circuits involved may not be able to compensate and deficits may be observed.

This is likely what was happening with Participant X as he drove and tried to find his car. Behaviours that involve executive functioning are abundant in everyday life and contribute to the orchestration of goal-directed behaviour. Insult to this ability affects success. Participant X has not nailed down a full time job and he struggles to feel like a success. In the end, however, he shrugs and gives in to smoke a joint while I talk with him, unable to get past the apathy that marijuana seems to plague long term users with. Is this what we want for society?

....

References

Fried, P.A. 1995 "The Ottawa Prenatal Prospective Study (OPPS): Methodological Issues and Findings—It's easy to throw the baby out with the bath water". Life Sciences 56(23-24): 2159-2168

Fried, P. 2002 Adolescents prenatally exposed to marijuana: examination of facets of complex behaviors and comparison with the influence of in utero cigarettes. Journal of Clinical Pharmacology 42: 97S-102S

Fried, P.A., Watkinson, B., Gray, R. 1998 Differential effects on cognitive functioning in 9-12 year olds prenatally exposed to cigarettes and marihuana. Neurotoxicology and Teratology 20: 293-306

Fried, P.A., Watkinson, B., Gray, R. 2003 Differential effects on cognition functioning in 13-16 year olds prenatally exposed to cigarettes and marihuana. Neurotoxicology and Teratology 25: 427-436

Fried, P.A., Watkinson, B., Gray, R. 2005 Neurocognitive consequences of marihuana—a comparison with pre-drug performance. Neurotoxicology and Teratology 27(2): 231-239

Hatchard, T., Fried, P.A., Hogan, M.J., Cameron, I., Smith, A.M. (in press) Does regular marijuana use impact cognitive interference? An fMRI investigation in young adults using the Counting Stroop task. Journal of Addiction Research and Therapy

Smith, A.M., Longo, C., Fried, P.A., Hogan, M.J., Cameron, I. 2010 Effects of marijuana on visuospatial working memory: An fMRI study in young adults. Psychopharmacology 210(3): 429-438

Smith, A.M., Zunini, R.A.L., Anderson, C.D., Longo, C.A., Cameron, I., Hogan, M.J., Fried, P.A. 2011 Impact of marijuana on response inhibition: an fMRI study in young adults. Journal of Behavioural and Brain Sciences 1: 24-33

Andra Smith, Ph.D. is a Professor of Neuroscience in Ottawa. She is one of the only fMRI researchers in the region and continues to work on understanding the neural mechanisms of drug abuse, particularly marijuana use in youth. Her Ph.D. was completed at the University of British Columbia followed by a CIHR funded Post-doctoral fellowship at Carleton University. Her current position at the University of Ottawa began in 2004 and she continues as a tenured professor to educate youth on the significant negative impact of marijuana on the brain.

NATIONAL CANNABIS PREVENTION AND INFORMATION CENTRE
University of New South Wales, Australia

Mixing Cannabis and Alchohol

POLYDRUG USE IS using more than one drug at the same time. People use drugs in combination to either increase their intoxication, or to increase the effect of the first drug taken.

Sometimes people mix two drugs because they are already intoxicated and are no longer making rational decisions about their drug-taking and the wellbeing of themselves and those around them. The more drugs being used at the same time, the more likely it becomes that things will go wrong.

Not counting tobacco, the most common form of polydrug use is alcohol and cannabis. When people mix cannabis and alcohol together at one time, the results can be unpredictable. The effects of either drug may be more powerful, or the combination may produce different and unpredictable reactions.

What are the effects of mixing cannabis and alcohol?

When people smoke cannabis and drink alcohol at the same time they can experience nausea and/or vomiting, or they can react with panic, anxiety or paranoia. Mixing cannabis with alcohol can increase the risk of vulnerable people experiencing psychotic symptoms.

There is some evidence to support that having alcohol in your blood causes a faster absorption of THC (the active ingredient in cannabis that causes intoxication). This can lead to the cannabis having a much stronger effect than it would normally have and can result in 'greening out'.

Greening out is a term commonly referred to in a situation where people feel sick after smoking cannabis. They can go pale and sweaty, feel dizzy, nauseous and may even start vomiting. They usually feel they have to lie down straight away.

It appears that this is more likely to happen if a person has been drinking alcohol before smoking cannabis rather than the other way around.

What are the risks of mixing cannabis and alcohol?

- unpredictable effects—if cannabis and alcohol are used at the same time there is a greater likelihood of negative side effects occurring either physically (greening out) or psychologically (panic, anxiety and paranoia).
- effects on driving—the negative effect that alcohol has on driving is well documented.
- Cannabis use also affects a person's ability to concentrate

and react in driving situations. Even at low doses the combination of alcohol and cannabis is dangerous and places the drivers, their passengers and others on the road at serious risk.

- getting too intoxicated—making a person less aware of their surroundings and less likely to be able to maintain control of situations, for example, not being able to look after their belongings or to negotiate safe sex.
- substituting one drug for another—people trying to cut back on one drug may end up using more of the other to help manage the symptoms of reducing the first drug. For example, some people giving up cannabis may find it difficult to sleep and start drinking alcohol at night to help them sleep and vice-versa. This type of drug use is risky and can result in a person having problems with two drugs instead of one.

Reprinted with permission. *Factsheet*. National Cannabis Prevention and Information Centre.

ED WOOD
President DUID Victim Voices
Colorado, USA

An Open Letter to States Considering Legalization of Marijuana

THOSE WHO SAY that Colorado's "experiment" in legalizing marijuana proves it can be done safely with proper regulation don't realize that in an experiment, one must control input variables and measure outcomes. Colorado does neither, so its dalliance with legalization cannot properly be termed an experiment. Although it regulates retail and "medical" cannabis stores, the July 9th Department of Revenue report shows that less than one-half of Colorado's estimated 160 metric ton annual consumption of marijuana comes from regulated stores. And measuring outcomes? The only outcome that is measured by the state is tax revenue, which is falling short of projections.

Driving under the influence of drugs, including marijuana, has never been measured by Colorado. Like most states, Colorado has a single statute number for DUI, whether caused by alcohol, drugs, or a combination of the two. There is simply no mechanism to track drug impairment, much less marijuana impairment on a statewide basis.

Recognizing that problem, this year (2014) the Colorado State Patrol began a manual collection of DUI-marijuana data, based upon officer's beliefs about the cause of observed impairment. In six months, they wrote 349 citations for DUI where marijuana was believed to be a cause of impairment. Since the State Patrol issues less than 20% of the state's DUI citations, one might infer a DUI-marijuana prevalence of 3,500 annually.

Unfortunately, there are few tools available to detect and/or measure DUI-marijuana, so the estimate of 3,500 is likely understated. Unlike alcohol's impairment that is predominantly a physical impairment, marijuana's impairment is predominantly mental. Less than 2% of Colorado's officers are trained to recognize, document and testify to DUID based on symptoms unique to drug impairment. Standardized roadside tests designed to confirm alcohol impairment are only marginally successful identifying drug impairment, especially for chronic users.

For many reasons, blood tests that are so useful to confirm alcohol impairment are nearly useless to confirm marijuana impairment. Drugs or alcohol never impair blood, urine, or oral fluids. Only the brain is impaired. Blood testing is a surrogate for testing what's in the brain. For alcohol, it's a good surrogate; for drugs, much less so. There are three reasons for this:

1. The blood-brain barrier is more effective in slowing the transit of high molecular weight drugs than it is for low molecular weight alcohol, and drugs like THC remain in fatty tissues like the brain long after they are removed from the blood,
2. Individual responses to marijuana's impairing THC are less predictable than responses to alcohol, and
3. The average 2 hour time between a crash and a blood draw allows THC in the blood from smoked marijuana to decline by 90% or more, frequently below the limits of detection, even for someone who was smoking at the time of the crash.

Marijuana may be judged safer than alcohol because no one has died from taking marijuana. By that simplistic measure, it's also safer than the bubble gum that choked Michael Jones to death. But it's still not safe. Marijuana causes driving impairment, and it causes deaths such as Tanya and Adrian Guevarra, killed by a driver who confessed to driving under the influence of marijuana after testing positive for 4 ng/ml of Delta 9 THC.

Pot proponents ask to have marijuana regulated like alcohol. But it's not like alcohol. It's a drug, and its legalization as proposed does not serve the interests of public safety.

DUID Victim Voices performs research, education and lobbying in the field of drug-impaired driving. Drug use is considered by many to be a victimless "crime", yet those killed or injured by drug-impaired drivers demonstrate the simplicity of this argument.

Mr. Wood has worked with victims, prosecutors, defense attorneys, judges, clinicians, drug recognition experts, law enforcement officers, toxicologists, state officials, and an international list of researchers and other specialists in his quest to increase public knowledge about DUID. He has been an invited speaker on DUID topics for law enforcement, international research, and state agencies. In 2013 he was named an Advocate for Action by the President's Office of National Drug Control Policy. (http://www.whitehouse.gov/blog/2012/12/03/join-chorus-voices-speaking-out-against-drugged-driving)

His intense quest began four years ago, after the death of his 33-year old son Brian, two months before the birth of Brian's daughter. Brian and two others lost their lives at the hands of two drug impaired drivers on marijuana, methamphetamine and heroin. The women were charged with vehicular homicide due to driving under the influence of drugs. The defense attorney pointed out during trial, "It is not unlawful to drive with illegal drugs in your body." The two drivers were found guilty of vehicular homicide due to driving with disregard for the safety of others. Assuming normal parole, the drivers will serve only 18 months in prison per homicide.

He is a retired medical device executive who founded COBE BCT, Inc., now Terumo BCT, based in Colorado. Ed and his wife Janice live in Morrison, Colorado

MARY BRETT
Chair, CanSS, and Member of WFAD
UK

Cannabis: General Facts

An Extract from '*Cannabis: A General Survey of its Harmful Effects*'
Updated October 2014

CANNABIS SATIVA GROWS well in tropical and temperate climates. Marijuana consists of the dried plant parts, Hashish is the resin secreted by glandular hairs all over the plant mainly round the flowers, protecting the plant from water loss. Sinsemilla is the dried material from the tops of the female plants. Hashish oil (up to 60% THC), is obtained by extraction but rarely used in the UK.

Cannabis contains some 400 chemical substances. These vary with the habitat and are often contaminated with microbes, fungi or pesticides (Jenike 1993, BMA 1997). More than 60 cannabinoids, substances unique to the plant have been identified. The most psychoactive of these and the main cause of many of the other harmful pharmacological effects is THC (delta-9-tetrahydrocannabinol) (Ranstrom 2003). Other natural cannabinoids are delta-8-THC, cannabinol and cannabidiol (BMA 1998).

Brain signals pass along nerve cells in the form of electrical impulses, and chemicals called neurotransmitters carry the messages between cells. These dozens of neurotransmitters are released at the end of one neuron (nerve cell) and fit into receptor sites by shape on the next cell. Transmission of nerve signals takes a fraction of a second. The psychoactive THC mimics a neurotransmitter called anandamide and so affects its receptor sites (Devane et al, 1992).

Two types of receptor site have been identified, CB1 receptors are distributed in the brain in the areas concerned with motor activity and control of posture (cerebellum and basal ganglia), emotion (amygdala and hippocampus), memory, cognition, the "high", distortion of the sense of time, sound, colour and taste, the alteration of the ability to concentrate and the production of a dreamlike state (cerebral cortex and hippocampus), sensory perception (thalamus), mood in general and sleep. No CB1 receptors are present in the brain stem so the drug does not affect basal bodily functions like respiration. This explains the lack of deaths by overdosing with cannabis (Harkenham et al, 1991, 1992, BMA 1997). CB2 receptors were discovered in 1994 by Lynn and Harkenham. They were outside the brain on specific components of the immune system. Binding of cannabinoids was also seen in the heart, lungs, endocrine and reproductive systems, so all these systems are affected.

Cannabinoids are absorbed rapidly into the body after inhalation from smoked cannabis preparations. The effects become noticeable in a matter of minutes. They are then rapidly distributed all over the body and maximum brain concentrations are reached within 15 minutes. The psychological effects can last for 2 to 4 hours then slowly decline over the next 12 hours. When taken orally, THC absorption is much slower and more variable and the onset of its effects are delayed by 30 minutes to 2 hours. The duration of its effects are prolonged, 5 to 6 hours due to continued absorption from the gut and some cognitive and motor skills are impaired for much longer e.g. driving. (Huestis et al 1992, BMA 1997). Cannabis can cross the placenta, enter the circulation of the foetus and pass into breast milk.

Cannabinoids are highly lipid-soluble and so rapidly accumulate in the fatty tissues, being slowly released back into other body tissues and organs including the brain and bloodstream. Elimination of a single dose can take 30 days, unlike water-soluble alcohol which is removed at the rate of one unit per hour, and appears in the faeces and urine. Repeated doses will therefore accumulate in the body and affect the brain over long periods of time (BMA 1997). Cannabis is a multi-faceted drug. The inhibitory effects of THC on the release of a variety of neurotransmitters in the central nervous system has also been observed in several studies (Schliker and Kathmann, 2001, Katona et al 2000). Blood levels of THC drop rapidly after smoking due to its conversion into metabolites and sequestration into fatty tissues (Grotenhermen 2003).

Since 1971 when drugs were classified and cannabis was consigned to class B, the amount of THC in the plant in some varieties of Cannabis sativa has changed considerably. At that time the content of THC in marijuana was around 0.5–3% (Ranstrom 2003). Smokers in the late 80s and 90s had access to sensemilla (7 to 11% THC, Schwartz 1991). Hashish has consistently had a THC content of 4 to 5%. However, selective breeding of the plant, especially in Holland, has produced varieties such as Netherweed and Skunk with THC contents up to and over 20% (Jenike, 1993, BMA 1998).These stronger types, now commonly grown in the UK are favoured by today's users, the lower levels being much less common (Ranstrom 2003). An article in The Guardian on 29th August 2006 reported that "Analysis of recent home-grown hauls detected THC levels as high as 20%, nearly 7 times higher than samples of imported resin, which used to be the predominant form of the drug on the streets, and typically contained around 3% THC" Detective Inspector Neil Hutchison said, "A decade ago 11% of the cannabis sold on the street was grown in the UK. Now more than 60% is produced in Britain ... ". The Forensic Science Service, Drugs Intelligence Unit confirmed this figure (10/10/06) and said that between 30 and 40% of the rest is imported resin, some imported herbal cannabis is still seen as well. At a meeting of the Science and Technology Committee of the House of Commons on 22nd November 2006, Dr Brian Iddon MP said that 70% of the cannabis in the UK is home grown and is skunk. The discovery of a new high-potency hybrid known as "Colombian" in December 2006 in Mexico has sent alarm bells ringing. It can be planted at any time of year and matures in 2 months. Worse than that, it cannot be killed by pesticides. A plot the size of a football field yields as much as was formerly grown on a 10 to 12 acre plot (Associated Press, Mark Stevenson 20/12/06). A Home Office Cannabis Potency Study in 2008 found that seizures in early 2008 were 80.8% herbal and 15.3% resin, the rest (3.9%) were indeterminate or not cannabis. Over 97% of the herbal cannabis was sinsemilla (skunk), the remainder imported traditional. The mean potency of the sinsemilla was 16.2% (range 4.1 to 46%). The mean potency of the imported herb was 8.4% (range 0.3% to 22%) but accounted for very few samples. Mean potency of cannabis resin was 5.9%, similar to previous years. The CBD (antipsychotic) content of the herbal cannabis was less than 0.1% in nearly all cases. In the 60/70s herbal cannabis the CBD and THC content was almost equally balanced.

On 25th April 2007, the ONDCP (Office National Drug Control Policy) and NIDA (National Institute on Drug Abuse) issued the latest analysis from the University of Mississippi's Potency Monitoring Project that the highest ever levels of THC had been found since analysis began in the late 1970s. The average amount of THC in seized samples is 8.5%, up from 7% in 2003, in 1983 the average was under 4%. More than 60% of teens receiving treatment for drug abuse or dependence report marijuana as their primary drug of abuse. In 2005 the number of marijuana-related hospital emergency room admissions was 242,200 up from 215,000 in 2004. The highest concentration found in a sample was 32.3%. Roughly 60% of first-time marijuana users are under 18 in the USA.

Moir et al reported that cannabis smoke not only contains

about 50 substances that can cause cancer but also 20 times more ammonia (linked to cancer) than tobacco smoke. Hydrogen cyanide (linked to heart disease), nitrogen oxides (linked to lung damage) and certain aromatic amines were at levels 3 to 5 times more.

It should be mentioned that cannabis research is still very young. In 1996 the total number of scientific papers did not exceed 10,000 and today probably stands between 14 and 15,000. This is in contrast to research on tobacco with about 140,000 studies to date (Ranstrom 2003). The total collection of scientific papers on cannabis is held in the library of The University of Mississippi.

A new type of cannabis product was reported by Drug Watch International on 25th February 2008. It is called "Budder". It is reported as being the purest cannabis product available at anywhere between 82 and 99.6% pure THC/CBD/CBN. One hit is equalled to 1 to 2 full cannabis joints and the "high" to be clearer and more long-lasting than average marijuana. Inhalation is the method of choice. A miniscule amount (head of pin) is applied to heated metal and inhaled. Major effects usually subside in 3 to 4 hours, others up to 8 hours. Hallucinations, paranoia, disconnection and hunger can all be felt. It is extremely potent and its effects can be delayed, leading some users to 'over consume' and be overwhelmed. It is made by whipping in air and freezing isomerized hash oil. The delta –9-THC is converted to delta-6-THC so normally inactive cannabinoids are activated.

A paper in 2005 by Pijlman and others found a considerable

increase in the levels of THC in cannabis sold in Dutch coffee shops. In 2004, the average level of THC in home grown Dutch marijuana (Nederwiet) was 20.4%, significantly higher than that of imported marijuana at 7%. Dutch hashish (Nederhasi) contained 39.3% THC in 2004 compared with 18.2% in imported hashish. The average percentage of THC in Dutch marijuana, Dutch hashish and imported hashish had almost doubled since 1999. It had remained consistent in imported marijuana.

Another report into concentrations of THC in Dutch marijuana was conducted for 2009–2010 by The Netherlands Institute of Mental Health and Addiction (The Trimbos Institute). Random samples, sinsemilla (Nederwiet), imported marijuana, Dutch hash and hash from imported marijuana and the most potent herbal (202) were bought from coffee shops. The average THC content of all samples was 16.7%, and 22% in the hash samples. Average THC of Nederwiet was 17.8% imported marijuana 7.8%. Hash from Dutch hemp had more (32.6%) than hash from foreign cannabis (19.0%). Average THC in Nederwiet was higher in 2010 than 2009 (17.8 cf 15.1%). THC in foreign marijuana was lower than year before (7.5% in 2010 and 9.9% in 2009). Average most potent 17.9%. Nederwiet had considerably less CBD than imported marijuana.

The average THC content of skunk (over 80% of the UK market in 2008) was around 16%.

A new "form" of cannabis, SPICE (JWH-018), is being used by young people, and was legal in the UK. This is a synthetic psychoactive substance, created by an American academic purely for research purposes in 1995. According to The Royal Society of Chemists, it gives a "marijuana-like high" and is said to be 4 to 5 times stronger than THC. The chemical is added to packets of herbs, all legal. The structure of spice is quite different from THC but it has the same effects. It has already been banned in Holland, Austria, Germany and Switzerland. It was banned in the UK in December 2009.

In July 2010 Alexandra Datig found several very harmful fungi asssociated with marijuana. Black mould, Stachybotrys, exists on almost all building materials. The growth of cannabis indoors poses a great problem as it provids ideal conditions. Also the 3 most dangerous strains of Aspergillus, fumigitus, flavus and niger exist naturally on the plant. A deadly afla-toxin could be the result. A 1996 treatment study by Withenshawe Hospital, Manchester, on 10,000 patients with invasive Aspergillosis has shown $633m in costs, average $63,300/patient to treat not cure the disease.

In 2010, Arendt et al published mortality figures among 20,581drug users over a 10 year period (1996-2006) in Denmark. 1441 deaths were recorded in follow-up (111,445 person years). Standardised Mortality Ratios (SMRs) for primary users of specific substances were, cannabis 4.9, cocaine 6.4, amphetamine 6.0, heroin 9.1 and otheropioids 7.7. For ecstasy the crude mortality rate was 1.7/1000 person years.

In 1981, the WHO Report on Cannabis Use said, "It is instructive to make comparisons with the study of effects of other drugs, such as tobacco or alcohol. With these drugs, "risk factors" have been freely identified, although full causality has not yet been established. Nevertheless such risk factors deserve and receive serious attention with respect to the latter drugs. It is puzzling that the same reasoning is often not applied to cannabis" … "To provide rigid proof of causality in such investigations is logically and theoretically impossible, and to demand it is unreasonable".

March 2011 A S Reece published 'Chronic Toxicology of Cannabis.' 5198 papers were screened by hand and preferentially include the most recent ones.

Findings:

There is evidence of psychiatric, respiratory, cardiovascular, and bone toxicity associated with chronic cannabis use. Cannabis has now been implicated in the etiology of many major long-term psychiatric conditions including depression, anxiety, psychosis, bipolar disorder, and an amotivational state. Respiratory conditions linked with cannabis include reduced lung density, lung cysts, and chronic bronchitis. Cannabis has been linked in a dose-dependent manner with elevated rates of myocardial infarction and cardiac arrythmias. It is known to affect bone metabolism and also has teratogenic effects on the developing brain following perinatal exposure. Cannabis has been linked to cancers at eight sites, including children after in-utero maternal exposure, and multiple molecular pathways to oncogenesis exist.

Conclusion:
Chronic cannabis use is associated with psychiatric, respiratory, cardiovascular, and bone effects. It also has oncogenic, teratogenic, and mutagenic effects all of which depend upon dose and duration of use.

2011 Accidental poisoning in children was reported in 4 cases in a care centre in Southern Spain by Croche Santander B et al. Paediatric accidental cannabis poisoning is an uncommon but life-threatening intoxication. Reduced level of consciousness, drowsiness, ataxia, tremble, apnea, hypotonia and seizures were all witnessed. THC was detected by urine screening. All recovered and were discharged within 24 hours. They concluded that the possibility of cannabis poisoning should be considered in unexplained acute onset of neurological findings in previously healthy children.

Updated information on THC concentration in weed, netherweed and hash in Dutch coffee shops 2010 to 2011. Frans Koopmans, De Hoop Clinic, Dordrecht, Netherlands.

Since the nineteen seventies the policy on cannabis use in The Netherlands has substantially been different from that in many other countries. It is based on the idea that separating the markets for hard and soft drugs prevents cannabis users to resort to hard drug use. Over the years so-called coffee shops emerged. Coffee shops are alcohol free establishments where the selling and the use of soft drugs is not prosecuted, provided certain conditions are met. Many of the cannabis products sold in these coffee shops originate from Dutch-grown grass called 'Nederwiet'. On behalf of the Ministry of

Health, Welfare and Sports we investigate the potency of cannabis products as sold in coffeeshops in The Netherlands.

Δ^9-Tetrahydrocannabinol (THC) is the main psychoactive compound in marihuana and hashish. The aim of this study is to investigate the concentration of THC in marihuana and hash (=cannabis resin) as sold in Dutch coffee shops. In addition we examined whether there are differences between the cannabis products originating from Dutch grown hemp (nederwiet) and those derived from imported hemp. This is the twelfth consecutive year that this study has been performed. Apart from THC, the content of two other cannabinoids, cannabidiol (CBD) and cannabinol (CBN), are measured.

The names and addresses of 50 (out of a total of 666) Dutch coffee shops were randomly selected. For the purpose of this study, 65 samples of nederwiet, 19 samples of imported marihuana, 9 samples of Dutch hash and 56 imported hash samples were anonymously bought in the selected coffeeshops. In addition, 49 samples of the most potent (herbal) marihuana product available were bought. As a rule samples of 1 gram were bought. Samples were bought anonymously.

Traditionally hash contains more THC than marijuana. The average THC-content of all the marihuana samples together was 15,3% and that of the hash-samples 16,5%. The average THC-content of nederwiet (16,5%) was significantly higher than that of the imported marihuana (6,6%). The average THC-percentage of the marihuana samples that were bought as most potent (17,0%) did not differ from that of the most popular varieties of nederwiet (16,5%). Hash derived from Dutch hemp contained more THC (29,6%) than hash originating from foreign cannabis (14,3%). The average THC-percentage of nederwiet was lower in 2011 than in 2010 (16,5 vs. 17,8%), but this difference was not statistically significant. The THC-percentage in imported hash was significantly lower than the year before (14,3% in 2011 versus 19,0% in 2010).

There is some evidence that not only THC-content is indicative for the effects and risks of cannabis, but that CBD might attenuate some of the negative effects of THC. This means that cannabis with a high CBD / THC ratio would have less negative health consequences than cannabis that has little or no CBD. Nederwiet has very low levels of CBD (median = 0,3%), whereas imported hash contained on average 6,7% CBD.

The ratio between CBN and THC can give an indication of the freshness of the preparation (Ross and Elsohly, 1997). Levels of CBN were higher in imported marihuana and hash compared to products derived from homegrown cannabis. Also the ratio of CBN/THC was significantly higher in the imported products. The ratio was higher in imported marijuana compared to nederwiet and in imported hashish as compared to hashish made from nederwiet. Prices that had to be paid for imported marihuana were lower than those for any of the other cannabis products. The prices of hash made from nederwiet were higher. The average price for a gram nederwiet increased from 2007 to 2009 (up to 50%), but since then prices remained the same. On average, a gram of nederwiet costs €8,30.

2012 Mason et al Treatment for cannabis addiction.

Gabapentin, on the market to treat neuropathic pain and epilepsy, helps people to quit marijuana use. 50 treatment –seeking users taking Gabapentin experienced fewer withdrawal symptoms, smoked less weed and scored higher on cognitive skills compared with those who had placebos. In the last 4 weeks of the study all Gabapentin users were cannabis free.

2012 Crippal and others looked at medicines to reduce intoxication (euphoria, disturbed perception, giggling, red eyes, dry mouth, increased appetite, increased heart rate,misperception of time etc). A recent increase in the number of emergency room visits for marijuana intoxication prompted researchers to look for medical treatment. Propanolol used to treat cardiac conditions reduced several symptoms in well-done studies.

2012 Simonetto et al investigated cannabinoid hyper-emesis in 98 patients who met the inclusion criteria ie recurrent vomiting and no other explanation but that of cannabis use. All were under 50—most had used cannabis for 2 years and more than once/week. Abdominal pain was common and hot baths/showers provided almost universal relief. They concluded, 'Cannabinoid hyper-emesis should be considered in younger patients with long-term cannabis use and recurrent nausea, vomiting and abdominal pain'.

2013 Kiriski looked at age of first time use of alcohol and cannabis to a transmissible risk for addiction in childhood and development of alcohol use disorder (AUD) and cannabis use disorder (CUD). They found that whereas transmissible risk is comparable to both AUD and CUD, its magnitude is 7 times greater in youths who initiated substance use with cannabis. The earlier they started, the greater the risk.

2013 Chueh et al looked at factors involved in the resistance of substance abuse. They found that 'being female', having strong knowledge about the substance, and negative attitude towards substance use correlated with higher levels of self-confidence to resist substance use.

2013 Bostwick found that medical marijuana use for pain may interfere with normal development. 3 high school age patients attended Mayo Clinic's chronic pain clinic. They were using cannabis for severe pain after everything else had failed. They reported worsening of the pain and impaired functioning. All 3 dropped out of school and social lives.

2013 Wang and others found no admissions of children under 12 for marijuana ingestion at a Colorado children's hospital before September 30th 2009, but 14 afterwards. 9 had lethargy, 1 ataxia, 1 respiratory insufficiency—8 were admitted, 2 to intensive care. Eight of the 14 cases involved medical marijuana and 7 of these exposures were from food products.

2013 Harrison et al looked at chronic non malignant pain in adolescents. 3 cases of using medical marijuana were studied. None relieved the pain. They concluded that … 'even short-term marijuana use may be associated with health and cognitive concerns that may prevent adolescents from achieving their full academic and vocational potential'.

2013 Chittamma et al found that umbilical cord tissue was a viable specimen for the detection of maternal use of marijuana.

2013 Hurd et al looked at the effects of cannabis through generations of male inheritance. Metabolic and behavioural effects of cannabis in rats during adolescence were passed down to multiple generations of male offspring, even though these animals were not themselves exposed to the drug.

2013 Wu and others found that cannabis use disorders (CUD) are comparatively prevalent among non-white racial/ethnic groups and adolescents in the USA. In USA, non-white population is growing faster than the whites. All confounding issues were controlled for. Compared with whites, mixed-race people had higher incidences of CU (Cannabis Use), Asian Americans and Hispanics had a lower incidence. Past-year cannabis users who were black, Native American, Hispanic or Asian American had higher odds of CUD than whites, in all ethnic groups—adolescents had higher odds than adults. Major depressive episodes, arrest history, nicotine dependence, alcohol disorder, were all associated with CU and CUDs. CUD disproportionately affects non-white groups and adolescents.

2013 Yetisan et al looked at Holographic Diagnostics in Medicine. 'Smart' holographs are used to detect various substances (including drugs) by turning colour in their presence. They are being researched at Addenbrooke's Hospital in Cambridge. In the presence of of certain compounds, the hydrogels either shrink or swell, causing the holograph to change colour. The process is fast, cheap and easy to use.

2013 Heron et al looked at prior cannabis risk factors and use at 16. Over 4,000 children provided information at the age of 16 in The Avon Longitudinal Study of parents and

Children. They found that cannabis use was more common in girls than boys, 21.4% v 18.3%. Problem cannabis use in boys was higher than girls, 3.6% v 2.8%. Early onset persistent conduct problems were strongly associated with problem cannabis use, odds ratio (OR) 6.46. Residence in subsidised housing, OR 3.10, maternal cannabis use, 8.84, any maternal smoking in the post natal period 2.69, all predicted problem cannabis use. Attributable risks for adolescent problem cannabis use associated with the previous factors were 25, 13, 17 and 24% respectively.

2013 Huang and others looked at adolescent substance use and obesity in young adulthood. 5141 adolescents were taken from the child sample of the 1979 National longitudinal Survey of Youth and biennial data across the 12 assessments from 1986 to 2008 was used. Cigarette smoking, alcohol use and marijuana use from age 12 to 18 and obesity trajectories from ages 20-24 were examined. Adolescents with the most problematic smoking trajectory, and those with an increasing marijuana trajectory were most likely to exhibit an increased obesity trajectory in young adulthood.

2014 Vallee et al discovered that Pregnenolone can protect the brain from cannabis intoxication. Pregnenolone is the inactive precursor of all steroid hormones. THC substantially increases the synthesis of pregnenolone in the brain via activation of the CB1 receptor. Pregnenolone then acting as a signalling specific inhibitor of the CB1 receptor reduces several effects of THC. This negative feedback protects the brain from CB1 receptor over-activation. This may open an approach for the treatment of cannabis intoxication and addiction.

2014 Wolff K Smoking infrequently a single cannabis cigarette leads to peak plasma concentrations of 21-267 micrograms/litre causing acute intoxication. Daily users the plasma THC concentrations are 1.0-11.0 micrograms/litre maintained by sequestration of the drug from the tissues.

2014 Hall and Degenhardt updated and summarised the most harmful effects of cannabis. They listed the most probable of the adverse health effects of regular cannabis use sustained over the years as indicated by epidemiological studies that have established the links. These are: dependence syndrome, impaired respiratory function, and cardiovascular disease, adverse effects on adolescent psychosocial development and mental health, and residual cognitive impairment.

2014 Hartung et al looked at cannabis as a cause of death. They conducted post-mortems on 15 people whose deaths were linked to cannabis use. Other factors that might have contributed to the death, alcohol, liver disease etc were discounted. Two of the deaths could not be attributed to anything else but cannabis intoxication. Both men died of cardiac arrhythmia triggered by cannabis, and had enough active THC in their blood to show they had taken it recently. Neither had a history of heart problems.

2014 Capretto warned parents of a new drug '10' times more potent than marijuana BHO, Butane Honey Oil, or Dab is made by extracting THC and the use of household items such as butane containers, glass or metal tubes, baking dishes and even coffee filters.

2014 April 2nd BBC News (Canada and US) reported the first death due to cannabis in Colorado since legalisation. An exchange student fell to his death after ingesting edible marijuana. A Post Mortem examination found marijuana intoxication was a factor in the death.

2014 Chheda et al found sleep to be affected by cannabis use. Results showed that any history of cannabis use was associated with an increased likelihood of reporting difficulty in falling asleep, struggling to maintain sleep, experiencing non-restorative sleep and feeling daytime sleepiness. The strongest association was found in those who started early, before 15 being about twice as likely to have severe problems, and to have sleep problems as adults.

2014 Danielsson et al found that heavy pot use in teen years may predict later-life disability. Those who smoked heavily at 18 were most likely to end up on the nation's (Sweden) disability rolls by 59. The Swedish cohort of 98% of the male population (conscripts) at baseline and a 39 year long follow up time provided new knowledge. Men who had used marijuana more than 50 times before the age of 18 were 30% more likely to go on disability sometime between 40 and 50 years of age.

2014 Volkow (NIDA) et al wrote an update on Adverse Health Effects of marijuana Use in The New England Journal of medicine

2014 Correspondence followed the article by Volkow and others.

....

References

Arendt M, Jorgensen P, Sher L, Jensen SO, Mortality among individuals with cannabis, cocaine, amphetamine, MDMA, and opioid use disorders: A nationwide follow-up study of Danish substance users in treatment. Drug Alcohol Depend. 2010 October22. (Epub ahead of print)

BMA *Therapeutic Uses of Cannabis* Harwood Academic Publishers 1997.

Bostwick JM, Marijuana and Chronic Nonmalignant Pain in Adolescents, Mayo Clinic Proceedings June 24th 2013.

Capretto Neil, Medical Director at Gateway rehab Pittsburgh. Feb 19th 2014

Chheda J, Grandner M, *Marijuana use Associated with impaired sleep quality.* American Academy of Sleep Medicine. ScienceDaily. ScienceDaily, 2 June 2014. <www.sciencedaily.com/releases/2014/06/140602102013.htm>.

Chittamma A, Marin SJ, Williams JA, Clark C, McMillin GA, Detection of *In-Utero* Marijuana Exposure by GC-MS, Ultra-Sensitive ELISA and LC-TOF-MS Using Umbilical Cord Tissue. J of Analytical Toxicology Advance Access July 10th 2013 1-4.

Correspondence re Volkow: http://www.nejm.org/doi/full/10.1056/NEJMc1407928

Crippal JAS, Derenusson GN, Chagas MHN, Atakan Z, et al, *Pharmacological interventions in the treatment of the acute effects of cannabis: a systematic review of literature* . Harm Reduction Journal 2012, 9:7 doi:10.1186/1477-7517-9-7 (January 2012)

Croche Santander B, Alonso Salas MT, Loscertales Abril M, *Accidental cannabis poisoning in children: report of four cases in a tertiary care center from Southern Spain.* Arch.Argent Pediatr 2011 Feb; 109(1): 4-7. 2013 Chueh et al looked at factors involved in the resistance of substance abuse. They found that 'Being female, having strong knowledge about the substance, and negative attitude towards substance use correlated with higher levels of self-confidennce to resist substance use.

Danielsson A-K (Karolinska Institute Sweden) et al, Heavy pot use in teen years may predict later-life disability, Drug and Alcohol Dependence August 2014

Datig A *Killer Fungus Grows on Marijuana* www.nipitinthebud2010.org

Devane WA, Hanus L, Breuer A et al Isolation and structure of a brain constituent that binds to the cannabinoid receptor Science 1992b; 258: 1946-9.

Drug Watch International. Feb 2008, Report of Budder. Cannabis promoting sites on the Internet all carry information about this product, e.g. Cannabis Culture and Cannabis World.

Grotenhermen F *Pharmacokinetics and Pharmacodynamics of Cannabinoids* Clin. Pharmacokinet 2003; 42(3): 327-60.

Hall W, Degenhardt L, *The adverse health effects of chronic cannabis use.* Drug test Anal 2014 Jan; 6(1-2):39-45. doi: 10.1002/dta. 1506 Epub 2013 Jul 8.

Harrison TE, Bruce BK, Weiss KE, Rummans MD, Bostwick MD, Marijuana and Chronic Nonmalignant Pain in Adolescents. Mayo Clinic Proc. July 2013: 88(7): 647-650.

Hartung B et al, Cannabis can kill without the influence of other drugs, Forensic Science International, DOI:10.1016/j.forsciint.2014.02.001 Herkenham M, Lynn AB, Johnson MR et al Characterization and Localization of Cannabinoid Receptors in Rat Brain: A Quantitative In Vitro Autoradiographic Study Journal of Neuroscience 1991; 11: 563-83.

Herkenham M Cannabinoid *Receptor Localization in Brain: Relationship to Motor and Reward Systems* Annals of the New York Academy of Sciences 1992; 654: 19-32.

Heron J, Barker ED, Joinson C, Lewis G, Hickman M, Munafo M, Macleod J, Childhood conduct disorder trajectories, prior risk factors and cannabis use at age 16: birth cohort study. Addiction. 2013 Dec; 108(12) :2129-38. doi: 10.1111/add.12268 Epub Jul 12.

Huang DY, Lanza HI, Anglin MD, Association between adolescent substance use and obesity in young adulthood: a group-based dual trajectory analysis. Addict. Behav. 2913 Nov; 38 (11): 2653-60. doi: 10.1016/j.addbeh.2013.06.024 Epub 2013 Jul3.

Huestis MA, Sampson AH, Holicky et al *Characterization of the Absorption Phase of Maruijuana Smoking* Clinical Pharmacology and Therapeutics 1992; 52: 31-41.

Hurd et al, Society for Neuroscience: Source reference: Hurd Y "Paternal cannabis exposure during adolescence reprograms offspring reward neurocircuitry in a sex-dependent manner" *SFN* 2013; Abstract 695.05. 2013

Jenike MA *Drug Abuse.* In Rubenstein E, Federmann DD (Eds) Scientific American Medicine, Scientific American Inc. 1993.

Katona I, Sperlagh B, Magloczky Z et al *GABAergic interneurons are the targets of cannabinoid actions in the human hippocampus* Neuroscience 2000; 100: 797-804.

Kiriski L, Tarer R, Ridenour T, Zhai ZW, et al, Age of alcohol and cannabis use onset mediates the association of transmissible risk in childhood and development of AUDs and CUDs: evidence for common liability. Exp Clin Psychopharmacol 2013 Feb: 21(1): 38-45. Epub Dec 2012.

Lynn AB, Herkenham M *Localization of Cannabinoid Receptors and Non-Saturable High-Density Cannabinoid Binding Sites in Peripheral Tissue of the Rat: Implications for Receptor-Mediated Immune Modualtion by Cannabinoids* Journal of Pharmacology and Experimental Therapeutics 1994; 268: 1612-23.

Mason BJ, Crean R, Goodell, Light JM, et al, *Concept Randomised Controlled Study of Gabapentin: Effects on Caanabis Use, Withdrawal and Executive Function Deficits in Cannabis-Dependent Adults.* Europsychopharmacology advance online publication 29th February; doi: 10.1038/npp.2012.14

Moir D et al, *Marijuana snmoke contains higher levels of Certain Toxins than Tobacco Smoke.* American Chemical Society Dec 18th 2007.

Morgan C, Curran HV, Effects of cannabidiol on schizophrenia-like symptoms in people who use cannabis. The British Journal of Psychiatry (2008) 192, 306–307. doi: 10.1192/bjp.bp.107.046649

Pijlman FTA, Rigter SM, Hoek J, Goldscmidt HMJ, Niesink RJM, *Strong increase in total delta-THC in cannabis preparations sold in Dutch coffee shops.* Addiction Biology June 2005; 10: 171-80.

Ranstrom J *Adverse Health Consequences of Cannabis Use: A survey of scientific* studies *published up to and including the autumn of 2003.* National Institute of Public Health, Sweden 2003.

Reece AS *Chronic Toxicology of Cannabis* Clin Toxicol (Phila) 2009 Jul;47(6):517-24.

Report of an ARF (Addiction Research Foundation)/WHO scientific meeting on adverse health and behavioural consequences of Cannabis Use, Toronto, Ontario. Alcoholism and Drug Addiction Research Foundation, Toronto 1981.

Schliker E, Kathmann M *Modulation of transmitter release via presynaptic cannabinoid receptors* Trends Pharmacol. Sci. 2001; 22: 565-72.

Schwartz RH *Heavy Marijuana Use and Recent Memory Impairment* Psychiatric Annals; 1991;21(2): 80-2.

Simonetto DA, Oxentenko AS, Herman ML, Szostek JH, Cannabinoid Hyperemesis : A Case Study of 98 Patients. Mayo Clinic Proc. Feb 2012:87(2) 114-119.

Vallee M, Bellocchio L, Hebert-Chatelain E, Monlezun S, Martin-Garcia E, et al, Pregnenolone can protect the brain from cannabis intoxication. Science 2014 January 3;343(6166):94-8.doi: 10.1126/science.1243985

Volkow ND, Baler RD, Compton WM, Weiss SRB, Adverse Health Effects of Marijuana Use. N Engl J Med 2014; 370:2219-2227June 5, 2014DOI: 10.1056/NEJMra1402309

Volkow correspondence: http://www.nejm.org/doi/full/10.1056/NEJMc1407928

Wang GS, Roosevelt MD, Heard K, Pediatric Marijuana Exposures in a Medical Marijuana State. JAMA Pediatr 2013; (): 1-4. doi 10.1001/jama-pediatrics. 2013.140.

Wolff K, Johnston A, Cannabis use: a perspective in relation to the proposed drug driving legislation. Drug Test Anal. 2014 Jan; 6(1-2): 143-54 doi: 10.1002/dta. 1588. Epub. 2013 Dec.

Wu LT, Brady KT, Mannelli P, Killeen TK, NIDA AAPII Workgroup. Cannabis use disorders are comparatively prevalent among non-white racial/ethnic groups and adolescents: A National study. J. Psychiatr. Res 2013 Dec pil: S0022-3956(13)00360-9. doi:10.1016/j.psychires.2013.11.010 (E=pub ahead of print).

Yetisan AK, Butt H, Vasconcellos F da C, Montelongo Y, Davidson C, Blyth J, Chan J, Carmody JB et al, Light-directed Writing of Chemically Tunable Narrow-Band Holographic Sensors. Advanced Optical materials 2013 DOI: 10. 1002/adom.201300375

Mary Brett is a retired biology teacher. She taught in a mixed comprehensive school in Glasgow for 5 years, then in an English Grammar school (selective) for boys for over 30 years where she was in charge of Health Education.

She has campaigned against cannabis for well over 20 years and is now Chair of the drug prevention charity, CanSS (Cannabis Skunk Sense, www.cannabisskunksense.co.uk. CanSS provides the admin for the APPG (All Party Parliamentary Group) on Cannabis and Children in the United Kingdom's House of Commons. She is also a member of WFAD (World Forum Against Drugs) and an ex-Vice President of Eurad.

MELDON KAHAN MD CCFP, SHERYL SPITHOFF MD CCFP
Women's College Hospital
Toronto, Ontario, Canada

How Physicians Should Respond to the New Cannabis Regulations

The Canadian Journal of Addiction

Note: Marijuana spelled two ways from Health Canada: 1) When referring to it in general terms "j"; 2) When referring to it in legal terms "h".

Abstract

The new Health Canada regulations on medical marihuana would allow patients to purchase dried cannabis from a licensed distributer with a medical prescription. Yet available evidence does not support the safety and efficacy of smoked cannabis as an analgesic. The controlled trials on smoked cannabis were very brief and had small sample sizes. The subjects had severe neuropathic pain syndromes, whereas most medical marihuana users have fibromyalgia, low back pain and other conditions commonly seen in primary care. None of these trials compared smoked cannabis to oral cannabinoids, which may be as or more effective than smoked cannabis for chronic pain. Oral cannabinoids are also far safer than smoked cannabis, which produces very high plasma THC levels, and toxic chemicals that are carcinogenic and atherogenic.

In addition, studies show that the population that uses medical marihuana for chronic pain is at higher risk for cannabis-related harms. Compared to pain patients in primary care, medical cannabis users are more likely to be younger, male, and to have a history of addiction or mental illness. This puts them at high risk for cannabis related harms such as addiction, psychosis, depression, poor school and work performance, and motor vehicle accidents. It is unsafe to prescribe cannabis to such patients, and also often unnecessary, since the majority of medical cannabis users have benign pain conditions for which numerous effective and safe treatments are available.

We propose that, for patients who are at low risk of harms from smoked cannabis, physicians sign a declaration rather than a prescription. A cannabis prescription endorses the therapeutic use of a substance which lacks medical evidence of benefit, and is much less safe than existing treatments. In contrast, a declaration affirms that the physician does not oppose, on medical grounds, the patient's decision to use a substance from which he or she at low risk of harm. Thus, a declaration maintains honesty and integrity in our interactions with our patients, directs physicians' attention towards assessment and intervention for cannabis-related harms, and encourages patients and physicians to consider other treatments, ones with proven benefit.

How Physicians Should Respond to the New Cannabis Regulations

The new Health Canada regulations on medical marihuana,

which go into effect in March 2014, would allow patients to purchase dried cannabis from a licensed distributer with a signed medical prescription. the official newspaper of the Government of Canada (1) describes the prescription as follows: 'The medical document would contain information similar to that on a prescription. The authorized health practitioner would have to indicate their licence information, the patient's date of birth and name, location of the assessment, and amount of dried cannabis authorized per day, for a period of up to one year.'

Both the Canadian Medical Association and the Federation of Medical Regulatory Authorities of Canada have expressed concern about the regulations. In a news release, Dr Anna Reid, president of the Canadian Medical Association, stated (2):

"Asking physicians to prescribe drugs that have not been clinically tested runs contrary to their training and ethics ... Patients would not want us to prescribe drugs for heart disease, cancer or any other illness without the scientific evidence to back those drugs up. Why does the federal government want us to do so with marihuana?"

The College of Family Physicians of Canada has issued a position statement in opposition to the proposed regulations (3):

"In our view, Health Canada places physicians in an unfair, untenable and to a certain extent unethical position by requiring them to prescribe cannabis in order for patients to obtain it legally ... Physicians cannot be expected to prescribe a drug without the safeguards in place for other medications—solid evidence supporting the effectiveness and safety of the medication, and a clear set of indications, dosing guidelines and precautions ..."

A prescription indicates that the physician believes that the medication will be safe and beneficial for the patient if taken as directed. Physicians can have confidence in their prescriptions, because Health Canada has reviewed the evidence on the medication's safety and effectiveness, and has approved its therapeutic use for the indications and at the doses stated in the drug monograph. Yet Health Canada has not approved smoked cannabis for therapeutic use, and the available evidence on safety and effectiveness falls far short of the standards it uses to approve other prescription medications.

Efficacy of Smoked Cannabis as an analgesic

To date, according to the 2013 Health Canada information bulletin on cannabis (4), five controlled trials have examined smoked cannabis in the treatment of chronic pain (5-9). These trials do not support making cannabis available as a prescription analgesic. All five trials enrolled subjects with neuropathic pain due to HIV, multiple sclerosis, or surgery. Yet observational studies have shown that medical marihuana users have similar diagnoses to the primary care pain population—fibromyalgia, back pain and arthritis (10). Participants were administered smoked cannabis for periods of between one to fifteen days, which is far too brief a period to detect potentially serious long-term side effects or to demonstrate improvements in functional capacity, which is the most important outcome of analgesic trials. Furthermore, the total sample of the five trials was 182, and subjects smoked cannabis under tightly controlled, artificial conditions.

To illustrate how weak this evidence is, a 2006 metaanalysis of opioid analgesic medications reviewed 41 controlled trials, involving over 6,000 subjects, with a mean trial duration of 5 weeks (11). Multiple opioid trials have been conducted on common primary care conditions such as osteoarthritis and low back pain. Despite this, the long-term safety and effectiveness of opioids remains a topic of considerable controversy.

Of equal concern, none of the trials compared smoked cannabis to currently available cannabinoids, ie oral nabilone (Cesamet) or the buccal spray (Sativex). Smoking delivers THC to the central nervous system more quickly and efficiently than oral ingestion. However, higher plasma levels are not necessarily associated with better pain control. In a study of capsaicin-induced pain, volunteers reported reduced pain with a 4% cannabis cigarette, and increased pain with an 8% cigarette (12). In the only controlled study (to our knowledge) that directly compared smoked to oral cannabis (14), subjects administered the cold pressor test had equal intensity but shorter duration of analgesia with smoked cannabis than with oral dronabinol. This result is not surprising, since oral cannabinoids are metabolized to an active metabolite, 11-hydroxyTHC, which prolongs the duration of analgesia (4).

Safety of smoked cannabis

Not only is smoked cannabis possibly less effective than oral cannabinoids, it is also far less safe. The difference in peak plasma levels between smoked cannabis and oral cannabis are striking. An average peak THC plasma level of 162 ng/ml is reached after smoking seven puffs of a 3.55% THC cigarette (4). In contrast, a standard 2 mg dose of oral nabilone produces a peak plasma concentration of 10 ng/ml. The onset of action of smoked cannabis is 30 seconds, whereas nabilone's onset of action is 30 minutes. In other words, compared to a 2 mg nabilone tablet, a single low-potency joint has an onset of action 60 times faster and a peak plasma level 16 times higher than a 2 mg nabilone tablet. The THC concentrations associated with euphoria are only 50-100 ng/mL, or 1.5-3 times lower than that produced by a single joint (4). And these figures underestimate the plasma levels produced by current street cannabis, which has average THC concentrations of 10% (4).

The controlled studies do not provide information on the long term safety of smoked cannabis because of their short duration, but the limited evidence available is not reassuring. A systematic review of adverse events in trials on medical cannabis (15) found a higher rate of non-serious adverse events in the intervention group, including psychiatric events. However, studies on smoked cannabis were excluded from this review because they did not adequately report data on adverse events. Also, the median duration of the studies was only two weeks. Another systematic review of 18 controlled trials on both smoked and oral cannabis (16) estimated that the odds ratio and numbers needed to harm (NNH) for three adverse reactions were as follows: alterations to perception, OR 4.51, NNH 7; altered motor function, OR 3.93, NNH 5; and altered cognitive function, 4.46, NNH 8. In the long term, these adverse reactions could lead to serious complications such as trauma and impaired work performance.

Besides the acute and chronic effects of intoxication, smoking creates hundreds of toxic products of combustion. Some of these products are carcinogenic Epidemiological studies on the association between smoking cannabis and various types of cancer have had conflicting results (4). However, a recently published study provides the strongest epidemiological evidence to date that smoked cannabis is a risk factor for lung cancer. In this 40-year retrospective cohort study of 50,000 Swedish male conscripts, regular cannabis smoking was associated with a 2-fold risk of lung cancer, even after controlling for tobacco use and other factors (42). Smoking also creates byproducts that are atherogenic and may precipitate angina or myocardial infarction (23).

The byproducts of combustion can be minimized by mixing cannabis in food, or by 'vaporizing' cannabis (heating the dried plant until the cannabis on the plant's surface vaporizes). A preliminary study (17) demonstrated that vaporizing produces much lower concentrations of exhaled carbon monoxide than smoking. However, while vaporization and oral ingestion are probably safer than smoking, physicians who prescribe the dried cannabis plant cannot control how the patient uses the cannabis, and smoking remains the most popular delivery route.

Long-term harms of smoked cannabis

Of greater concern is the risk cannabis prescribing presents to higher risk patients. Evidence suggests that medical cannabis users are at higher risk than the general pain population for cannabis addiction and other harms, because they tend to be young and male (established risk factors), and they have higher rates of concurrent mental illness and concurrent opioid and illicit drug misuse. A study of 457 fibromyalgia patients attending a tertiary care pain center (19) found that patients who used cannabis were more likely to be male and had significantly higher rates of current unstable mental illness and opioid drug-seeking behavior compared to patients who did not use cannabis. A systematic literature review found that chronic pain patients on opioids have a higher prevalence of aberrant opioid-related behaviours if they use cannabis than if they do not (20). Another study found that chronic pain patients who had a positive urine drug screen for cannabis were much more likely to have a positive UDS for cocaine (21). Prescribing cannabis to such patients puts them at risk for mental illness, addiction, poor school and work performance, accidents, and other serious harms (see section below).

Conversely, if physicians decline to prescribe cannabis to higher risk patients, it may create tension in the patient-physician relationship. This situation already exists with prescription opioids. In a random survey of primary care physicians in Ontario (22), 57.6% of physicians reported they were somewhat or very concerned about disagreements with patients over opioids.

Medical Cannabis policy and public health

It is important to distinguish the impact of policies on medical marihuana from social policies on legalization or decriminalization. National drug policies that emphasize strict enforcement instead of prevention, harm reduction and treatment are clearly harmful. Portugal, recognizing this, decriminalized possession of cannabis and other illicit drugs in 2002. While drug trafficking remains a criminal offense, drug possession is an administrative offense resulting in fines, community service or referral to treatment. Portugal's policy has been associated with a marked decline in the use of cannabis and other drugs, and in drug-related harms such as overdose and infection (13). In contrast, in the US, states which allow the use of marihuana for medical purposes have higher rates of cannabis use, and cannabis dependence, than states which do not authorize it (18). This may be because states which allow medical marihuana also tend to have more liberal attitudes to cannabis use.

This demonstrates that a increasing access to medical marihuana provides none of the social benefits of decriminalization. It does not protect young cannabis users from incarceration, and it does not promote prevention, harm reduction or treatment. On the contrary, making smoked cannabis available by prescription reinforces the public's perception that it is harmless, which could increase cannabis use and cannabis-related harms. The dramatic increases in opioid overdose deaths and addiction rates reflect, in part, the public's perception that opioids must be safe if they are so widely prescribed by doctors.

As well, increasing access to smoked medical marihuana without addressing the wider prohibition of cannabis makes little sense as public policy. The large majorit of cannabis smokers do not have chronic pain and will thus remain vulnerable to criminal charges. Medical prescriptions will likely increase cannabis use and cannabisrelated harms in high-risk patients, and could well give a significant boost to the illicit drug market.

Declaration versus a prescription

We propose that physicians sign a declaration rather than a prescription (Table 1). The declaration would state that the patient has a medical condition requiring treatment, and that the patient believes that medical marihuana relieves these symptoms. The declaration would further state that the patient is not, to the physician's knowledge, suffering from or at high risk for cannabis-related harms. It would also state that the patient has been informed of the risks of cannabis use, and of alternative therapies for his or her medical condition. We also recommend that patients be required to sign a document indicating that they understand that the declaration is not a prescription and that the physician does not necessarily endorse their use of cannabis (Table 3).

There are several advantages to this approach. Unlike a prescription, a declaration does not mean that the physician has directed the patient to smoke cannabis as a treatment for the patient's medical condition. It merely affirms that this particular patient is at low risk for harms related to cannabis use. And physicians will be able to focus on managing the patient's chronic pain, without ongoing disagreements about cannabis prescriptions. This is similar to a physician discussing alcohol use with a patient whose alcohol consumption is within the low risk drinking guidelines. The physician is not advising the patient to drink, but is simply offering an opinion that the patient's alcohol consumption does not pose a high risk for harm.

The declaration does not contain all the elements of a prescription. For example, it does not specify the amount of dried cannabis authorized per day, and it does not list the physician's medical licence number. Therefore it might not be sufficient to authorize the licensed cannabis distributor to sell cannabis to the patient. This is an issue for Health Canada to rectify. Health Canada cannot expect physicians to sign prescriptions for smoked cannabis without first approving it for therapeutic use, and specifying its indications, dose and precautions.

If Health Canada refuses to accept a declaration in lieu of a prescription, then we recommend that only physicians with a special license be authorized to write a cannabis prescription. To obtain such a license, physicians should be required to pass a training course, organized by a national medical organization. Cannabis distributers would only be authorized to dispense cannabis for prescriptions signed by physicians with a cannabis license. This would be similar to the Health Canada authorization for prescribing methadone for pain. Physicians with a special cannabis licence would be expected to prescribe it only for evidence-based indications, such as intractable vomiting, anorexia caused by cancer or HIV, or severe HIV neuropathy. Even with these conditions, oral or buccal cannabinoids should be tried first.

The most important advantage of a declaration over a prescription is that it directs physicians' attention towards assessment and intervention for cannabis-related harms. While most people smoke cannabis without any evidence of harm, for some it poses a major health hazard. Physicians can play an important role in identifying and intervening with such patients, just as they do with alcohol and other substances.

Low risk cannabis use

Low risk use of cannabis is not as well defined as low risk use of alcohol. Therefore these recommendations may change as more research is conducted. As well, the daily dose of THC used by a patient is difficult to estimate because of wide variations in inhalation patterns and in the weight and THC content of cannabis "joints".

Physicians should screen all patients who request medical marihuana for a cannabis use disorder, and for factors that put them at risk for developing a cannabis use disorder. Risk factors include a younger age, current or past problem with cannabis or other substances, and an active mental illness. Patients who are at high risk for developing a cannabis use disorder should be advised to use cannabis with caution, and to avoid daily use. They should not be given a declaration for smoked marihuana. Patients with an active cannabis use disorder should be offered counselling (27), follow-up, and possibly medication to relieve withdrawal symptoms and cravings (31). Those who are not able to reduce or quit should be offered a referral to an addiction medicine physician and a psychosocial treatment program.

Another group at high risk of harm are those with a current, past or family history of psychosis. Cannabis use is a well established risk for psychosis and for the development of schizophrenia (25). This group should be advised to abstain completely from cannabis, and should not be prescribed cannabis in any form.

Although a causal relationship has not been established, cannabis use is associated with mood and anxiety disorders, and an increased risk of suicide in both psychotic and non-psychotic samples (32,35). Patients with active mood and anxiety disorders or suicidal ideation should be counseled to reduce or abstain from any cannabis use.

Oral cannabinoids are likely safer for patients with cardiovascular or respiratory illness. Patients who decline oral forms and continue to smoke marihuana should be advised to use a vaporizer. If they continue to smoke, they should be advised to avoid tobacco, and to avoid deep inhalation and breath-holding.

Women who are pregnant, planning to become pregnant or at high risk for unplanned pregnancies should be counseled not to use cannabis. Preliminary evidence links maternal cannabis use to subtle neurodevelopmental abnormalities in infants (28).

And finally the under 25 population appears to be a very vulnerable group. The age at which cannabis use becomes safer is unclear; some sources suggest 18, some 21, others 25. While the life-time prevalence of cannabis dependence among regular smokers is estimated to be 9% (36), a substantially higher proportion of regular adolescent smokers report symptoms of dependence (41), and early cannabis use is associated with problematic use of other illicit drugs (34,38,39). Besides substance use disorders, adolescent users appear to be at risk for long-term cognitive impairment, social dysfunction, impaired work and school performance, anxiety and depression, and psychotic disorders (25, 26,30,37,40). And finally this population is the most likely to ride in a vehicle with a driver under the influence of cannabis. Cannabis use prior to driving increases the risk of accidents (29).

A recent publication reviewed these harms and has proposed lower risk use guidelines (summarized in Table 2). This publication occurred before the publication of the 2012 study that demonstrated the persistent 8 point IQ drop in adolescents who smoked marihuana regularly (33). Physicians should provide all patients who use or are considering the use of smoked cannabis with information on how to lower their risk of harm.

Conclusion

There is not enough evidence to support the safety and effectiveness of smoked cannabis as an analgesic. Oral cannabinoids may be more effective than smoked cannabis for chronic pain, and are almost certainly safer. Many medical cannabis users are also at high risk for cannabis related harms, including mental illness, addiction, poor work and school performance, and trauma. Prescribing cannabis to such patients will increase their risk of serious harm. Furthermore, most medical cannabis users have common pain conditions for which there are effective and safe treatments.

We propose that physicians sign a declaration rather than a prescription. The declaration would state that the patient is not suffering from or at high risk for cannabis related harms, and that the physician has informed the patient of the risks of cannabis use. The declaration affirms that the patient is at low risk for harm from cannabis use is not likely to cause serious harm. The declaration maintains honesty and integrity in our interactions with our patients as it does not endorse a medically unestablished treatment. Additionally, the declaration directs physicians' attention towards assessment and intervention for cannabis-related harms; evidence suggests that medical cannabis users are at greater risk for cannabis addiction and other harms than the general pain population. If Health Canada is unwilling to change the new regulations, then cannabis prescribing should be restricted to physicians who have completed a training course.

TABLE 1: *Sample Physician Declaration*

I declare that:

- This patient has a medical condition requiring treatment.
- The patient reports that cannabis relieves the symptoms caused by this medical condition.
- To my knowledge, the patient is not suffering from, and is not at high risk for, harms related to cannabis.
- The patient has been informed of the potential risks of medical cannabis
- The patient has been informed of alternative therapies for the patient's medical condition.

Table 2: *Recommendations to minimize the risk of cannabisrelated harms (adapted from Fischer et al, reference 24)*

Cannabis use should be delayed until early adulthood (eg 18+ years).
Users should not use cannabis daily, and should avoid or limit their use of higher-potency cannabis products.
Frequent users who experience problems related to cannabis use and/or have difficulty controlling their use should attempt to abstain, and if necessary should seek professional help.
Use vaporizers rather than smoking joints, blunts or water pipes.
If unwilling to stop smoking, avoid smoking cannabis with tobacco, and avoid deep inhalation or breath-holding.
Do not drive for at least 3-4 hours after use (longer if larger doses are used or acute impairment persists).
The following groups should abstain from cannabis use: • Pregnant women • Middle-aged or older patients with cardiovascular illness • Individuals with a history of psychosis, or a firstdegree relative with a history of psychosis.

TABLE 3: *Sample informed consent document for patients to sign*

1. I understand that this declaration does not imply that my physician has advised me to use medical cannabis. I will not hold my physician liable for any harms I might suffer as a result of my cannabis use.
2. My physician has informed me of the health risks associated with smoked cannabis.
3. My physician has informed me of alternative medical treatments available for my condition.
4. I understand that the risk of harm increases with the amount smoked, and that vaporization and oral ingestion of cannabis may be less harmful than smoking.
5. I promise not give or sell medical cannabis to others, as this is both illegal and dangerous.
   Signed: ________________Date: ___________
   Witness: _______________________________

Reprinted with permission. *Canadian Journal of Addiction*. Volume 4 Number 3 September 2013. Pages 13–20.

References

1. The Canada Gazette, Dec 15 2012
2. Laura Eggertson, Canadian Medical Association Journal 109, p 4528, June 27, 2013. NEWS: "New medical marihuana regulations shift onus to doctors to prescribe"
3. The College of Family Physicians of Canada. Statement on Health Canada's Proposed Changes to Medical Marihuana Regulations, February 2013
4. Controlled Substances and Tobacco Directorate at Health Canada, February 2013. Information for Health Care Professionals: Cannabis (marihuana, marihuana) and the cannabinoids.
5. Abrams D. I., Jay C. A., Shade S. B., Vizoso H., Reda H., Press S. et al. Cannabis in painful HIV-associated sensory neuropathy: a randomized placebocontrolled trial, Neurology 2007; 68: 515-521.
6. Wilsey B., Marcotte T., Tsodikov A., Millman J., Bentley H., Gouaux B. et al. A randomized, placebo-controlled, crossover trial of cannabis cigarettes in neuropathic pain, The journal of pain: official journal of the American Pain Society 2008; 9: 506-521.
7. Ellis R. J., Toperoff W., Vaida F., van den Brande G., Gonzales J., Gouaux B. et al. Smoked medicinal cannabis for neuropathic pain in HIV: a randomized, crossover clinical trial, Neuropsychopharmacology : official publication of the American College of Neuropsychopharmacology 2009; 34: 672-680.
8. Corey-Bloom J., Wolfson T., Gamst A., Jin S., Marcotte T. D., Bentley H. et al. Smoked cannabis for spasticity in multiple sclerosis: a randomized, placebo-controlled trial, CMAJ : Canadian Medical Association journal = journal de l'Association medicale canadienne 2012; 184: 1143-1150.
9. Ware M. A., Wang T., Shapiro S., Robinson A., Ducruet T., Huynh T. et al. Smoked cannabis for chronic neuropathic pain: a randomized controlled trial, CMAJ : Canadian Medical Association journal = journal de l'Association medicale canadienne 2010; 182: E694-701.
10. Aggarwal S. K., Carter G. T., Sullivan M. D., ZumBrunnen C., Morrill

R., Mayer J. D. Characteristics of patients with chronic pain accessing treatment with medical cannabis in Washington State, Journal of opioid management 2009; 5: 257-286.

11. Furlan A. D., Sandoval J. A., Mailis-Gagnon A., Tunks E. Opioids for chronic noncancer pain: a meta-analysis of effectiveness and side effects, CMAJ : Canadian Medical Association journal = journal de l'Association medicale canadienne 2006; 174: 1589-1594.
12. Wallace M., Schulteis G., Atkinson J. H., Wolfson T., Lazzaretto D., Bentley H. et al. Dose-dependent effects of smoked cannabis on capsaicin-induced pain and hyperalgesia in healthy volunteers, Anesthesiology 2007; 107: 785-796.
13. Greenwald, G. Drug decriminalization in Portugal: Lessons for creating fair and successful drug policies. White paper report for CATO Institute, April 2, 2009.
14. Cooper Z. D., Comer S. D., Haney M. Comparison of the analgesic effects of dronabinol and smoked marihuana in daily marihuana smokers, Neuropsychopharmacology: official publication of the American College of Neuropsychopharmacology 2013; 38: 1984-1992.
15. Wang T., Collet J. P., Shapiro S., Ware M. A. Adverse effects of medical cannabinoids: a systematic review, CMAJ : Canadian Medical Association journal = journal de l'Association medicale canadienne 2008; 178: 1669-1678.
16. Martin-Sanchez E., Furukawa T. A., Taylor J., Martin J. L. Systematic review and meta-analysis of cannabis treatment for chronic pain, Pain medicine (Malden, Mass) 2009; 10: 1353-1368.
17. Abrams D. I., Vizoso H. P., Shade S. B., Jay C., Kelly M. E., Benowitz N. L. Vaporization as a smokeless cannabis delivery system: a pilot study, Clinical pharmacology and therapeutics 2007; 82: 572-578.
18. Cerda M., Wall M., Keyes K. M., Galea S., Hasin D. Medical marihuana laws in 50 states: investigating the relationship between state legalization of medical marihuana and marihuana use, abuse and dependence, Drug and alcohol dependence 2012; 120: 22-27.

19. Ste-Marie P. A., Fitzcharles M. A., Gamsa A., Ware M. A., Shir Y. Association of herbal cannabis use with negative psychosocial parameters in patients with fibromyalgia, Arthritis care & research 2012; 64: 1202-1208.
20. Reisfield G. M., Wasan A. D., Jamison R. N. The prevalence and significance of cannabis use in patients prescribed chronic opioid therapy: a review of the extant literature, Pain medicine (Malden, Mass) 2009; 10: 1434-1441.
21. Pesce A., West C., Rosenthal M., West R., Crews B., Mikel C. et al. Marihuana correlates with use of other illicit drugs in a pain patient population, Pain physician 2010; 13: 283-287.
22. Wenghofer E. F., Wilson L., Kahan M., Sheehan C., Srivastava A., Rubin A. et al. Survey of Ontario primary care physicians' experiences with opioid prescribing, Canadian family physician Medecin de famille canadien 2011; 57: 324-332.
23. Singla S., Sachdeva R., Mehta J. L. Cannabinoids and atherosclerotic coronary heart disease, Clinical cardiology 2012; 35: 329-335.
24. Fischer B., Jeffries V., Hall W., Room R., Goldner E., Rehm J. Lower Risk Cannabis use Guidelines for Canada (LRCUG): a narrative review of evidence and recommendations, Canadian journal of public health = Revue canadienne de sante publique 2011; 102: 324-327.
25. Fergusson D. M., Horwood L. J., Swain-Campbell N. R. Cannabis dependence and psychotic symptoms in young people, Psychological medicine 2003; 33: 15-21.
26. Fergusson D. M., Horwood L. J., Swain-Campbell N. Cannabis use and psychosocial adjustment in adolescence and young adulthood, Addiction (Abingdon, England) 2002; 97: 1123-1135.
27. Fischer B., Jones W., Shuper P., Rehm J. 12-month follow-up of an exploratory 'brief intervention' for high-frequency cannabis users among Canadian university students, Substance abuse treatment, prevention, and policy 2012; 7: 15.
28. Wong S., Ordean A., Kahan M. Substance use in pregnancy, Journal of

obstetrics and gynaecology Canada : JOGC = Journal d'obstetrique et gynecologie du Canada : JOGC 2011; 33: 367-384.

29. Mann R. E., Adlaf E., Zhao J., Stoduto G., Ialomiteanu A., Smart R. G. et al. Cannabis use and self-reported collisions in a representative sample of adult drivers, Journal of safety research 2007; 38: 669-674.

30. Dragt S., Nieman D. H., Schultze-Lutter F., van der Meer F., Becker H., de Haan L. et al. Cannabis use and age at onset of symptoms in subjects at clinical high risk for psychosis, Acta psychiatrica Scandinavica 2012; 125: 45-53.

31. Levin F. R., Mariani J. J., Brooks D. J., Pavlicova M., Cheng W., Nunes E. V. Dronabinol for the treatment of cannabis dependence: a randomized, double-blind, placebo-controlled trial, Drug and alcohol dependence 2011; 116: 142-150.

32. Serafini G., Pompili M., Innamorati M., Rihmer Z., Sher L., Girardi P. Can cannabis increase the suicide risk in psychosis? A critical review, Current pharmaceutical design 2012; 18: 5165-5187.

33. Meier M. H., Caspi A., Ambler A., Harrington H., Houts R., Keefe R. S. et al. Persistent cannabis users show neuropsychological decline from childhood to midlife, Proceedings of the National Academy of Sciences of the United States of America 2012; 109: E2657-2664.

34. Lynskey M. T., Vink J. M., Boomsma D. I. Early onset cannabis use and progression to other drug use in a sample of Dutch twins, Behavior genetics 2006; 36: 195-200.

35. Cheung J. T., Mann R. E., Ialomiteanu A., Stoduto G., Chan V., Ala-Leppilampi K. et al. Anxiety and mood disorders and cannabis use, The American journal of drug and alcohol abuse 2010; 36: 118-122.

36. Danovitch I., Gorelick D. A. State of the art treatments for cannabis dependence, The Psychiatric clinics of North America 2012; 35: 309-326.

37. Degenhardt L., Coffey C., Romaniuk H., Swift W., Carlin J. B., Hall W. D. et al. The persistence of the association between adolescent cannabis use and common mental disorders into young adulthood, Addiction (Abingdon, England) 2013; 108: 124-133.

38. Fergusson D. M., Boden J. M., Horwood L. J. Cannabis use and other illicit drug use: testing the cannabis gateway hypothesis, Addiction (Abingdon, England) 2006; 101: 556-569.

39. Fischer B., Rehm J., Irving H., Ialomiteanu A., Fallu J. S., Patra J. Typologies of cannabis users and associated characteristics relevant for public health: a latent class analysis of data from a nationally representative Canadian adult survey, International journal of methods in psychiatric research 2010; 19: 110-124.

40. Horwood L. J., Fergusson D. M., Coffey C., Patton G. C., Tait R., Smart D. et al. Cannabis and depression: an integrative data analysis of four Australasian cohorts, Drug and alcohol dependence 2012; 126: 369-378.

41. Nocon A., Wittchen H. U., Pfister H., Zimmermann P., Lieb R. Dependence symptoms in young cannabis users? A prospective epidemiological study, Journal of psychiatric research 2006; 40: 394-403.

42. Callaghan R. C., Allebeck P., Sidorchuk A. Marihuana use and risk of lung cancer: a 40-year cohort study, Cancer causes & control : CCC 2013 Jul 12. PubMed PMID: 23846283. Epub 2013/07/13. Eng.

"Big Marihuana Lobby Fights Legalization Efforts - Byron Tau." POLITICO. Accessed August 20, 2013. http://www.politico.com/story/2013/07/bigmarihuana- lobby-fights-legalization-efforts-94816.html.

"War on Drugs: REPORT OF THE GLOBAL COMMISSION ON DRUG POLICY JUNE 2011." REPORT OF THE GLOBAL COMMISSION ON DRUG POLICY, June 2011. http://www. globalcommissionondrugs.org/wp-content/ themes/gcdp_v1/pdf/Global_Commission_Report_English.pdf.

Dr. Meldon Kahan is the Medical Director of Addictions Medicine Service at St. Joseph's Health Centre's Mental Health & Addictions Program and an associate professor and funded researcher in the Department of Family and Community Medicine at the University of Toronto. In 2008 he was awarded the President's Shield for his outstanding contribution to the field of addictions in Ontario. Dr.Kahan is a member of the advisory council of SAM Canada.

Sheryl Spithoff MDm CCFP Women's College Hospital, Toronto, Ontario, Canada

PAMELA MCCOLL
Director and Advisory Council Member to Smart Approaches to Marijuana Canada

Marijuana and Pregnancy: What Are the Risks?

THE PUBLIC DISCUSSION and debate over marijuana, both as a recreational drug and for medicinal use, rages on. Negotiating through the rhetoric has left many of us searching for an objective, evidence based discussion. In the context of maternity and marijuana there are specific, recent scientific findings that can assist in making appropriate choices for the well-being of mother and child. We now have solid scientific findings that demonstrate that marijuana is not harmless, but a potent drug that can cause harm to the brain maturation in the fetus. It is critically important to understand the science of marijuana use in pregnancy to protect both mother and child.

Marijuana use during pregnancy interrupts fetal brain development. This can result in permanent damage and compromise the development of future cognitive abilities (1). It is the tetrahydrocannabinol (THC), the active ingredient in marijuana, that impacts the growth of the brain and this stage of the brain's development. Research conducted at the Icahn School of Medicine at Mount Sinai Hospital in New York, along with studies at the Medical University of Vienna and the Karolinska Institute in Stockholm, demonstrated that fetuses exposed to cannabis showed significantly lower levels of the protein needed for the development of cognitive abilities required to conduct planning, memory, decision making and organization functions.

Pregnant women need to know of the risks associated with marijuana use on the fetal brain and if they are using this drug either recreationally or for a relief of nausea associated with morning sickness. Smoking marijuana during pregnancy has been shown to decrease baby's birth weight, most likely due to the effects of carbon monoxide on the developing fetus (2). According to Dr. Andra Smith, Associate Professor at the University of Ottawa, School of Psychology: Yes, it might make the morning sickness subside but at what cost? The long term consequences may well be far more damaging than the short term relief. Marijuana crosses the placental barrier and has subtle effects on the newborn baby. However, it is the longer lasting and more delayed effects on cognitive processing that are most alarming. The prenatal exposure to cannabis contributes to a vulnerability of neurocognitive functioning that has been observed as early as 3 years of age and most strikingly continuing into young adulthood.

The growing evidence for a negative impact of prenatal cannabis exposure originates from three longitudinal studies worldwide. Due to the wide range of lifestyle variables that contribute to both brain, body and mental health, prospective studies are required to ensure control of as many of these variables as possible. This is the methodology that has been used for the Ottawa Prenatal Prospective Study (OPPS; 9) in Canada, the Maternal Health Practices and Child Development Project (MHPCDP; 10) in the US and the Generation R study in Europe (11).

Each of these studies investigated prenatal marijuana exposure in varying samples with different testing measures, and for these reasons all results are not comparable. However, the significant results that are consistent across the OPPS and MHPCDP, the two studies that have tested children for the longest period of time, and include neurocognitive challenges in the areas of short-term memory, as well as verbal outcomes, aspects of attention, impulsivity and abstract visual skills (9,10,12,13). These deficits appear after age 3 and continue into young adulthood (14,15). Most significantly, at 6 years of age, children exposed prenatally to marijuana showed more impulsive and hyperactive behaviour. This continued into adolescence and was accompanied by problems in abstract and visual reasoning, as well as visuo-perceptual functioning. These are the types of skills required to perform "top down processing", such as good decision making, organizing behaviour, setting goals and putting into action a plan to accomplish the goals. Each of these cognitive processes can be grouped under the umbrella term of executive functioning.

Executive functioning is required for success in life,

including schooling, relationships and work life. Struggles can occur in these facets when executive functions are compromised, something that can occur with prenatal marijuana exposure (16). Regular use during pregnancy is cause for concern.

In summary, prenatal marijuana exposure does have negative consequences on both the mother and child. This impact should be known so that expectant mothers can make informed choices about how to treat their morning sickness and ultimately care for the future of their children.

....

References

[1] Giedd, J.N. (2004). Structural magnetic resonance imaging of the adolescent brain. Annals of the New York Academy of Sciences. 1021, 77-85.

[2] Hall, W. & Degenhard, L. (2009). Adverse health effects of non-medical cannabis use. Lancet. 374, 1383-1391.

[3] Tetrault, J.M. (2007). Effects of cannabis smoking on pulmonary function and respiratory complications: a systematic review. Archives of Internal Medicine. 167, 221-228.

[4] Hoffman, D., Brunnemann, K.D., Gori, G.B. & Wynder, E.E.L. (1975). On the carcinogenicity of marijuana smoke. In: V.C. Runeckles, Ed., Recent Advances in Phytochemistry. New York: Plenum.

[5] Moore, T.H., Zammit, S., Lingford-Hughes, A. et al., (2007). Cannabis use and risk of psychotic or affective mental health outcomes: A systematic review. Lancet. 370 (9584), 319-328.

[6] Large, M., Sharma, S., Compton, M., Slade, T. & Nielssen, O. (2011). Cannabis use and earlier onset of psychosis: a systematic meta-analysis. Archives of General Psychiatry. 68(6), 555-561.

[7] Arseneault, L., Cannon, M, Poulton, R., Murray, R., Caspi, A., & Moffitt, T.E. (2002). Cannabis use in adolescence and risk for adult psychosis: longitudinal prospective study. British Medical Journal. 325, 1212-1213.

[8] Wagner, F.A., & Anthony, J.C. (2002). From first drug use to drug dependence; developmental periods of risk for dependence upon cannabis, cocaine, and alcohol. Neuropsychopharmacology. 26, 479-488.

[9] Fried, P.A. (1982). Marihuana use by pregnant women and effects on offspring: an update. Neurotoxicology and Teratology. 4, 451-454.

[10] Goldschmidt, L., Day, N.L., Richardson, G.A. (2000). Effects of prenatal marijuana exposure on child behavior problems at age 10. Neurotoxicology and Teratology. 22, 325-336.

[11] Jaddoe, V.W.V., van Duijn, C.M., Franco, O.H., van der Heijden, A.J. et al., (2012). The Generation R Study: design and cohort update 2012. European Journal of Epidemiology. 27, 739-756.

[12] Fried, P.A. Watkinson, B. (2000). Visuoperceptual functioning differs in 9-12 year olds prenatally exposed to cigarettes and marijuana. Neurotoxicology and Teratology 22, 11-20.

[13] Richardson, G.A., Ryan, C., Willford, J et al., (2002). Prenatal alcohol and marijuana exposure: effects on neuropsychological outcomes at 10 years. Neurotoxicology and Teratology. 24, 309-320.

[14] Smith, A.M., Fried, P., Hogan, M., Cameron, I. (2006). Effects of prenatal marijuana on visuospatial working memory: An fMRI study in young adults. Neurotoxicology and Teratology. 28, 286-295.

[15] Smith, A.M., Fried, P., Hogan, M., Cameron, I. (2004). Effects of prenatal marijuana exposure on response inhibition: An fMRI study of young adults. Neurotoxicology and Teratology. 26(4), 533-542.

[16] Fried, P.A. & Smith, A. (2001). A literature review of the consequences of prenatal marihuana exposure: an emerging theme of a deficiency in aspects of executive function. Neurotoxicology and Teratology. 23, 1-11.

Pamela McColl, has been working in the field of publishing for two decades. In 2012 McColl published the first ever smoke-pipe-free edition of the famous holiday poem *'Twas the Night Before Christmas*—capturing global media attention including AP, The Colbert Report, NBC Nightly News and the BBC. She is the author of *Baby and Me Tobacco Free* (2013). McColl is a director and advisory council member for SAM Canada (www.samcanada.net), and a board member on the Campaign for Justice on Tobacco Fraud. En.wikipedia.org/wiki/Pamela_Mccoll

MARY BRETT
Chair, CanSS, and Member of WFAD

Cannabis and the Reproductive System, Pregnancy and Development of Children

(An Extract from *Cannabis: A General Survey of its Harmful Effects*)

In the mid-seventies animal experiments suggested that cannabis adversely affects the secretion of gonadal hormones in both males and females, and the foetal development of animals given THC during pregnancy (Bloch 1983, Nahas 1984, Nahas and Frick 1987, Wenger et al 1992).

Research was triggered by the reporting of gynecomastia (breast development) in 3 young men (23 to 26) all heavy cannabis users (Harmon 1972). These findings are now in doubt as a small case-controlled study failed to find a relationship in 11 cases and controls (Cates and Pope 1977), and Mendelson (1984) said there would surely be more cases as the number of young men using cannabis was high.

Kolodny and others investigated men who were chronic cannabis users in 1972. They had reduced plasma concentrations of testosterone, sperm count and motility, with an increased number of abnormal sperm. Bloch 1983, Wenger 1992, and The National Academy of Science 1982, gave support to all his findings with experiments on animals.

Wenger said they were either due to the action of THC on the testes and/or the brain hormones that stimulate sperm production.

Kolodny's results were contradicted by Mendelson and others in 1974 in a large well-controlled study of heavy users. Other studies have produced positive and negative findings of the effect of THC on testosterone.

Although the reductions in testosterone and sperm numbers observed in some studies may not be of great significance in healthy adults, Hollister (1986) argued that they could pose problems in pre-pubertal males. A boy of 16, smoking cannabis since the age of 11, suffered from retarded development of the secondary sexual characteristics and growth. Partial recovery was attained 3 months after stopping (Copeland et al 1980). Also men with already impaired fertility may be at risk.

Dr Lani Burkman of Buffalo University Medical School, New York, reported to the annual meeting of The American Society of Reproductive Medicine in San Antonio, Texas on October 13th 2003. She had looked at the sperm of 22 frequent cannabis users (14 times a week for at least 5 years) and compared it with that of 59 men, non-users who had children. She found that the sperm were moving too fast, too soon. They would "burn out" before they reached the egg and would be unable to fertilise it. She suggested this may be a cause of infertility. She also found the users produced fewer sperm.

Studies on female fertility have also produced conflicting results. Bloch found that on exposing non-pregnant animals to THC, there was interference with the hormones concerned in reproduction produced in the brain. Oestrus was delayed, as was ovulation by a reduction of luteinising hormone and an increase in prolactin secretion. Rozenkrantz (1985) said exposure of pregnant women to THC was too risky as it may damage the foetus. Conflicting results have also been obtained on the cycling of sex hormones and duration of menstrual cycles in women.

The blastocyst stage of the embryo has to be implanted in the uterus wall for its continued development. Anandamide, the neurotransmitter mimicked by THC is produced at a high level in the uterus before implantation and then down-regulated at the time of implantation. High levels of anandamide induce spontaneous pregnancy loss in women. The use of cannabis at this crucial time during pregnancy may have the same effect (Paria et al 2001, Wang et al 2003).

A paper in 2006 (Klonoff-Cohen et al) on the effects of marijuana use on the outcomes of IVF (In Vitro Fertilisation) and GIFT (Gamete Intra-Fallopian Transfer) fertility treatments found that the prospect of a good outcome is reduced if either of the partners uses marijuana. Females produced fewer eggs and the child had a significantly lower birth weight, the more recent the use, the worse the effects. Male marijuana use was also associated with lower birth weight. Both timing and amount of the drug used negatively affected IVF and GIFT.

The risk of miscarriage or ectopic pregnancy of women

smoking cannabis in the early stages of pregnancy was highlighted in recent research by Dey and others in 2006. Anandamide controls the development of the embryo so the level of the neurotransmitter is crucial. THC by mimicking anandamide disrupts the correct signaling process. The embryos of mice treated with THC had more cell abnormalities than the controls and the embryos failed to travel to the uterus.

THC passes through the placenta in animals and humans, so it could potentially damage the embryo (Bloch 1983, Blackard and Tennes 1984). It is also passed in breast milk (Astley and Little 1990).

Experiments on animals have shown a number of very serious effects on gestation of offspring born to females given THC during pregnancy. These results must lead to a consideration of the possibility of similar effects occurring in humans (Abel 1985). In another paper in 1985 Abel found that a combination of alcohol and marijuana caused 73% fetomortality (offspring deaths) in rats and 100% in mice.

There is now consistent evidence to show that habitual cannabis smoking during pregnancy is associated with a lower than average birth weight (Hatch and Bracken 1986, Zuckerman et al 1989, Sherwood et al 1999) and height (Zuckerman et al 1989 and Tennes 1985) the relationship persists after control for confounding variables. Gibson and his colleagues in 1983 looked at the cases of 36 women, using cannabis 2 or more times/week. Twenty five per cent of them had premature births. An increased risk of prematurity was also found by Sherwood et al 1999.

Earlier experiments before the mid-eighties, not surprisingly produced inconsistent results as they were often conducted with insufficient care.

In 1995 Shiono and others failed to find any significant association between marijuana smoking and birth weight, however when the mothers blood was tested a clear tendency towards lower birth weight was apparent.

An analysis of 10 different studies into the effects of cigarette smoking in 1997, 7 of which involved cannabis use, displayed only a weak association between cannabis use and birth weight. For any use of the drug the average reduction was 48g. Use 4 times a day averaged 131g loss of weight. They concluded that the difference was small compared to the effects on birth weight of tobacco smoking, and that there is inadequate evidence that cannabis at the amount typically consumed by pregnant women, causes low birth weight (English et al 1997).

There are enormous problems in conducting surveys of this type. Heavy use of cannabis during pregnancy is rare, many samples are too small (Greenland et al 1982a/b, Fried 1980). Because of its illegality, many women are unwilling to be honest about their drug taking so lots of them will be classed as non-drug users (Zuckerman et al 1989). They are also likely to use alcohol, tobacco and other illegal drugs and tend to belong to a different social class (Fried, 1980, 1982, Tennes 1985). But the greatest problem is small numbers.

In 2002 the Avon Longitudinal Study of Parents and Children team in Bristol (Fergusson et al) looked at 12000 mothers expecting single babies. On average the babies were 216g lighter for women smoking once a week, they were significantly shorter and had smaller heads. When other factors were taken into consideration the average reduction in weight dropped to 90g. They equated the effect of a weekly joint to that of 15 cigarettes.

In animals very high doses of marijuana were needed to increase the rate of malformations occurring in the offspring. And indeed some experiments found this association (Linn et al 1983). Bloch (1983) found that in sufficient dosage, reabsorption, growth retardation and other malformations occurred in rats, rabbits mice and hampsters. But most of the best-designed studies failed to confirm these findings. Zuckerman et al in 1989 discovered among 202 infants, prenatally exposed to marijuana, a rate of malformations no higher than in a control group of non-using mothers. Gibson et al 1983, Hingson et al 1982 and Tennes et al 1985, uncovered no increase in the rate of major congenital abnormalities in children born to marijuana-using mothers.

Abel (1985) and Bloch (1983) suggested the malformations may be due to reduced nutrition due to the very high doses of the drug. Hollister (1986) added that "Virtually every drug that has ever been studied for dysmorphogenic effects has been found to produce these if the dose is high enough, enough species are tested or the treatment is prolonged".

However many of the papers that exonerate cannabis use were conducted using marijuana and not THC at the start of the eighties when the THC content of the marijuana widely used was very low. And Hall and others warned in 1994 that, "It would be unwise to exclude cannabis as a cause of malformation until larger and better-controlled studies have been carried out".

Malformations could of course be caused by chromosome damage. It has not been possible to show that THC can produce effects on specific genes which can cause abnormalities (Hall 1994, Hollister 1986). Cannabis smoke on the other hand is mutagenic (Bloch 1983). Hollister (1986) and The Institute of Medicine (1982) both discounted evidence that cannabinoids may cause mutations.

Three studies in the late eighties and early nineties linked cannabis use to an 11-fold increase in the cases of one form of leukaemia, ANNL (Acute Nonlymphoblastic Leukaemia) born to mothers using cannabis during pregnancy and increases in two other forms of childhood cancer, rhabdosarcoma and astrocytomas (Robison et al, 1989 Neglia al 1991, Grufferman et al 1993). The children with ANNL were younger than children with the disease born to non-using mothers and had cell differences which the researchers said made it unlikely that the relationship was due to chance.

There is little literature on the subject of the development of children whose mothers had smoked cannabis while pregnant. One study, unique in its longevity, The Ottawa Prenatal Prospective Study has been carried out from 1978 to the present day by Dr Peter Fried and his team. The children were examined neurologically immediately after birth and again several times in their first year. Tests for cognitive and psychomotor functioning were then executed yearly. At first, signs of neurological development deficiencies were detected, a delay in the development of the visual system and an increased rate of tremors and startle, as were withdrawal symptoms. These disappeared and nothing was reported till the age of four when memory and verbal ability were found to be deficient. At 5 and 6 these seemed to have gone but the six year olds had impaired ability to sustain attention.

From 6 to 9, several deficits in cognitive functions were noted and the parents reported behavioural problems. Between 9 and 12, there was a reduced ability as "regards memory in connection with visual stimuli, analytical ability and integrative ability". Again attention maintenance was a problem. The same pattern emerged from 13 to 16 (Fried 2003).

Fried et al in 1992 found that marijuana use increases the symptoms of ADHD in first grade children. Six year old children are more likely to show signs of this condition if their mothers smoked 6 or more marijuana cigarettes /week.

Fried said that the damage inflicted by cannabis at the foetal stage would not be noticed until the child needed to use his or her "executive" functions (for problem-solving and planning) at the age of four. Leavitt et al (1994) and Lundqvist (1995) found similar deficits in adult cannabis users. Fried also warns that the marijuana in 1978 when his investigation began had a much lower average THC content, so the risks may now be higher. On 15th July 2006 Dr Fried is due to give a talk at The 13th World Conference on Tobacco OR Health in Washington DC. As part of his long running study, he will say that children of mothers who smoked marijuana while pregnant are more than twice as likely to take up the habit when they reach adolescence.

Dahl (1995) had found sleeping problems in 3 year olds and Day (1994) lower intelligence scores also at the age of 3. These findings support those of Fried.

Another long-term study has been published. Goldschmidt and others in 2002 gathered data from over 250 women who used cannabis while pregnant. Reports from parents and teachers were used and at age 6 the teachers reported problems with delinquent behaviour. At 10, questionnaires were distributed and interviews conducted. A clear relationship between exposure to cannabis and delinquency was established, manifested by attention deficits, impulsiveness and hyperactivity.

Tennes and others in 1985 studied over 200 women who had used cannabis during pregnancy. The children were monitored after birth and again at one year old. They failed to find any differences between them and the controls.

An Italian research team under Vincenzo Cuomo (2003) injected pregnant rats with a low dose of artificial cannabinoid. The offspring were hyperactive. This disappeared at adulthood but was replaced by learning and memory retention problems. Because rats do not have confounding factors like tobacco smoking, standard of living or alcohol use, the results can be very useful. Fried said this showed great consistency with his study on humans.

The most recent study on the effects of pre-natal marijuana exposure (Day et al September 2006) has concluded that, " Prenatal exposure to marijuana , in addition to other factors, is a significant predictor of marijuana use at age 14". Other variables controlled for were: the child's current alcohol and tobacco abuse, pubertal stage, sexual activity, peer drug use, delinquency, family history of drug abuse and parental depression, current drug use, strictness and levels of supervision.

In 2002, Nahas and others reported that THC damages the formation of DNA in the dividing cells of testes and has been shown to impair the development of sperm cells in man. Marijuana or THC produces an early apoptosis of these fast-dividing cells and THC-induced apoptosis has also been found to occur in cells of the immune system (Zhu et al, 1998). Apoptosis is the "programmed cell death" of all our cells as they grow older, it is an irreversible biological process.

THC accumulates in fatty tissues and there are huge reserves of fat in the body for THC storage. With regular marijuana smoking the THC will build up quickly and take about 30 days to be completely eliminated. There will thus be a constant slow release of THC that will affect any processes going on in the body. Nahas concluded, " During chronic exposure to THC the pharmacokinetic molecular mechanisms which limit the storage of THC in the brain and testes are not sufficient to prevent a persistent deregulation of membrane signalling and the induction of functional and morphological changes which reflect a premature apoptosis of spermatogenic cells. Long-term longitudinal epidemiological studies have reported decreased spermatogenesis in healthy fertile adults".

Referring to 25-year old research findings on cannabis and the reproductive process detailed in his book *Marijuana and Medicine* 1999, Nahas said, "The latest studies in molecular biology have demonstrated that THC, the active ingredient in marijuana, damages the earliest stages of reproductive function. Thus marijuana is gametotoxic (toxic to embryos and sperm). It kills the reproductive cells of seven animal species, produces damage to the embryo, and retards foetal development. All of these destructive effects of marijuana on sperm cells, embryonic cells or lymphocytes have now been related to the early production of "apoptosis", the programmed death of the cell".

Frequent maternal marijuana use may be a weak risk factor for Sudden Infant Death Syndrome, SIDS (Scragg et al 2001).

In 2002 in The Princess Royal Maternity Hospital in Glasgow, drug tests (from the first stools) were carried out on 400 newly born babies. One in eight was found to have been exposed to cannabis in the womb. The study was carried out by forensic scientists from Glasgow University (Dr Ghada Abd-El-Azzim and Dr Robert Anderson), paediatric consultants (Lesley Jackson and Charles Skeoch) and senior registrar Scott Williamson. About 130 babies every year are treated at the hospital for drug dependency. Treatment can take days, weeks or months. According to the Forensic Science International Journal, more than 75% of babies exposed in this way will have medical problems later in childhood compared to 27% of the unexposed infants (Sunday Post 15/12/02).

A paper by Schuel et al in 2002 found evidence that anandamide signaling regulates human sperm functions required for fertilization. An analogue of AEA (anandamide) and also THC modulated capacitation and fertilizing potential of human sperm in vitro, sperm fertilizing capacity (in the Hemizonsa assay) was reduced by 50%. "These findings suggest that AEA-signaling may regulate sperm functions required for fertilization in human reproductive tracts, and imply that smoking of marijuana could impact these processes".

2002 Richardson and others looked at prenatal exposure to alcohol and marijuana and the effects on 10 year-old neuropsychological outcomes. At 10 over 500 children from a longitudinal study were tested for problem solving, learning, memory, mental flexibility, psychomotor speed, attention and impulsivity. Prenatal marijuana use had an effect on learning and memory as well as impulsivity.

2005 Gray et al looked at prenatal exposure and effects on depressive symptoms at age 10. 633 mother/child dyads were studied. Exposure to marijuana in the first and third trimesters predicted significantly increased levels of depressive symptoms (rather than a diagnosis of a major depressive disorder).

A review article was written in 2006 (Huizink and Mulder). They came to the conclusion; that pre-natal exposure to either maternal smoking, alcohol or cannabis use is related to some common neurobehavioural and cognitive outcomes, including symptoms of ADHD (inattention, impulsivity), increased externalising behaviour, decreased general cognitive functioning, and deficits in learning and memory tasks.

Bluhm et al in 2006 found that maternal recreational use of drugs and marijuana during pregnancy were associated with increased risk of neuroblastoma in offspring.

Barros and colleagues, writing in The Journal of Paediatrics in January 2007 found that marijuana-exposed infants born to adolescent mothers scored differently on measures of arousal, regulation and excitability compared to non-exposed infants, they showed subtle behavior changes in the first few days of life, they cried more, startled more easily and were more jittery. The authors said this may interfere with mother-child bonding.

Harkany et al in a paper in January 2007 found that endocannabinoid signaling modulates CNS (Central Nervous System) patterning so that "pharmacological interference with endocannabinoid signals during foetal development leads to long-lasting modifications of synaptic structure and functioning. Marijuana abuse during pregnancy can impair social behaviours, cognition and motor functions in the offspring with the impact lasting into adulthood.

Another paper in May 2007 had similar findings. Endocannabinoids in the human body play a vital role in the development of a baby's brain. They are responsible for controlling how the complex system of nerves develop in the embryonic brain. Dr Ann Rajnicek said "Smoking cannabis could interfere with the signals that are being used in the brain to wire it up correctly in the first place. As the brain develops further, there will be functional problems – potential brain damage" (Berghuis P et al 2007).

Forrester and Merz found selected birth defects with prenatal drug use in a study in Hawaii; December 2007. Cases were infants/fetuses with any one of 54 selected birth defects delivered during 1986-2002.

Marijuana rates were significantly higher than expected for 21(39%) of the birth defects. These defects were associated with the CNS, cardiovascular system, oral clefts, limbs and the gastrointestinal system.

A paper in March 2008 by Goldschmidt et al found that intelligence test performance was adversely affected at the age of 6 in children born to cannabis-using mothers. 648 children were involved in the study. Women were questioned about their use of marijuana at 4 and 7 months of pregnancy and at delivery. The results were: 'There was a significant nonlinear relationship between marijuana exposure and childhood intelligence. Heavy marijuana use (one or more cigarettes per day) during the first trimewter was associated with lower verbal reasoning scores on the Stanford-Binet Intellegence scale. Heavy use during the second trimester predicted deficits in the composite, short-term memory and quantitative scores. Third trimester heavy use was negatively associated with the quantitative score. Other significant predictors of intelligence include maternal IQ, home environment and social support'. They concluded that, "These findings indicate that prenatal marijuana exposure has a significant effect on school-age intellectual development".

2008 Aversa looked at erectile dysfunction in young habitual cannabis users. When cannabis is smoked, the arteries are constricted by a small amount. In long-term abusers, the arteries become so constricted that blood cannot properly flow to the penis. Men who chronically abuse marijuana show links to impotence since there is damage to the penile endothelium vasodilation and dilatation of brachial arteries. Dr. Aversa and his research team have concluded that, "early endothelial damage may be induced by chronic cannabis use (and endocannabinoid system activation)."

2008 April, Ian Russell, a specialist nurse practitioner in andrology and urology at Dumfries and Galloway Royal Infirmary in Scotland said, " In my clinic I see youngsters from the age of 17 onwards with sexual dysfunction. The age of onset of smoking cannabis is young, 10 years old in some areas. Puberty's kicking in and they're smoking regularly—5,6 joints a week. This can potentially suppress and traumatize the formation of leydig cells which secrete testosterone in the testes. This means these kids when they hit 14 or 15, will have sexual problems, for instance, not being able to get an erection, and possibly not having any sexual desire and a very very low testosterone level.

2008 Viagra is being prescribed for young men who use cannabis. The NHS in Scotland now spends £25m on Viagra, in some areas there is a 20% rise. There has been a rise in the number of teenage boys seeking help for erectile dysfunction.

Two experts have now linked this increase with cannabis use. Ian Russell, an expert on sexual health at Dumfries and Galloway Royal Infirmary, revealed more Scottish teens than ever before are suffering impotence after smoking cannabis during puberty, and Derek Rutherford, a specialist in sexual medicine for NHS Ayrshire and Arran, said he had prescribed Viagra to cannabis smokers.

I recently was in conversation with a midwife who had delivered babies of cannabis-using mothers. She said, "They are ravenous, chew their hands constantly, drink 3 times as much milk as non-affected babies, are promptly sick, then hungry again.

January 2010 El Marroun et al again found that maternal cannabis use even for a short period in pregnancy may be associated with lower birthweight and head circumference, and this this was more pronounced than the growth restriction seen in tobacco users. 7.5 thousand women were assessed.

2010 Gray et al: 86 pregnant women provided details of daily cannabis and tobacco use during pregnancy. Cannabis exposure was associated with decreased birth weight, reduced length and smaller head circumference, even after control for tobacco c-exposure.

2010 Campolongo et al looked at the developmental consequences of perinatal cannabis exposure neuroendocrine and behavioural effects in adult rodents.

Conclusions: 'There is increasing evidence from animal studies showing that cannabinoid drugs are neuroteratogens which induce enduring neurobehavioral abnormalities in the exposed offspring. Several preclinical findings reviewed in this paper are in line with clinical studies reporting hyperactivity, cognitive impairments and altered emotionality in humans exposed in utero to cannabis. Conversely, genetic, environmental and social factors could also influence the neurobiological effects of early cannabis exposure in humans'.

2010 Willford et al looked at prenatal tobacco, alcohol and marijuana, and their effects on processing speed, visual-motor coordination, and interhemispheric transfer. 320, 16-year olds, taking part in a longitudinal study into effects of prenatal substance exposure on development outcomes were investigated. No interactions were found between the 3 substances. Confounding factors were controlled for. There were significant and independent effects of the 3 on processing speed, and interhemispheric transfer of info. Tobacco and marijuana were implicated with deficits in visual-motor coordination.

2011 Shamloul reviewed the medical literature on cannabis use and sexual health. He revealed that cannabis use may negatively impact male sexual performance. While it was previously known that cannabis could affect certain receptors in the brain , it's now believed that these receptors also exist in the penis. Cannabis use may have an antagonizing effect on these receptors in the penis, making it more difficult for a man to achieve and maintain an erection.

2011 Day and others looked at the effects of prenatal marijuana exposure (PME) on delinquent behaviour. 580 mother/ child dyads were used from the 4th prenatal month through 14 years. Offspring of heavier marijuana users were significantly more likely to report delinquent behaviour at age 14. The odds ratio for delinquency for those exposed to one or more joints per day during gestation was 1.76. PME significantly predicted child depressive symptoms and attention problems at 10, after controlling for other significant covariants. Child depressive symptoms and attention problems at 10 significantly predicted delinquency at 14 years. The association between PME and delinquent behaviour at 14 years was mediated by depressive symptoms and attention problems in the offspring at 10 years.

2011 Frank et al studied the impact of intrauterine exposure to substances on initiation of use by adolescents. 149 adolescents who had been exposed to cocaine in the uterus were followed from birth till the age of 16. Higher levels of IUCE (intrauterine cocaine exposure) were associated with a greater likelihood of initiation of any substance (licit or illicit) as well as marijuana and alcohol specifically. Those with lighter intrauterine marijuana exposure had a greater likelihood of initiation of any substance as well as of marijuana particularly. Time dependent higher levels of exposure to violence between ages 8 and 16 were also robustly associated with initiation of any illicit or licit use and of marijuana and alcohol particularly.

2011 April: Marroun and others found, using stats from over 4000 children that intrauterine exposure to cannabis is associated with behavioural problems in early childhood with an increased risk for aggressive behaviour and attention problems as early as 18 months in girls, but not boys. No association was found between cannabis use of the father and child behaviour problems.

2011 Keimpema and others looked at the pre-natal development of the neuronal system. Endo-cannabinoid signalling orchestrates neuronal differentiation programs through timed interaction with the cannabinoid receptors. Cannabis, through prolonged switching on of these receptors high-jacks the system and leads to the erroneous wiring of neural networks. Cannabis-induced cannabinoid receptor activity over-rides physiological neuro-developmental endo-cannabinoid signals affecting the timely formation of synapses.

2012 Jan, Goldschmidt and others found, in a longitudinal study from birth, that a significant negative relation was found between prenatal exposure to marijuana (PME) and 14 year old WIAT(Wechsler Individual Achievement Test) composite and reading scores. The deficit in school achievement was mediated by the effects of PME on intelligence test performance at 6, attention problems and depression symptoms at 10, and early initiation of marijuana use.

Psychoyos et al in 2012 August found that new high-potency marijuana can interfere with early brain development in developing foetuses. 'Some new high-potency strains, including some medicinal cannabis blends , contain up to 20 times more THC than did 'traditional marijuana from decades past' said Delphine. Psychoyos, the co-author. 'Easy access to drugs via the internet or dispensaries makes the problem worse'. Harmful effects can begin as early as 2 weeks from conception. Exposure to today's marijuana in early pregnancy is associated with anencephaly, a devastating birth defect in which infants are born with large parts of the brain or skull missing.. Early pre-natal use was also tied up with ADHD. learning disabilities, memory problems in toddlers and 10 year olds as well as depression, aggression and anxiety in the teens.

Lacson and others in September 2012 found that marijuana use may increase the risk of developing subtypes of testicular cancer that tend to carry a worse prognosis. This result should be considered not only in people using cannabis recreationally but also when marijuana and its derivatives are used for therapeutic reasons in young male patients. 163 young men diagnosed with testicular cancer were compared with 292 healthy men of the same age and race/ethnicity. The marijuana-using men were twice as likely to have subtypes called non-seminoma and mixed germ cell tumours. These cancers usually occur in younger men and carry a worse prognosis than the seminoma type. These results confirm those of 2 previous studies of marijuana and testicle cancer.

2013 Fiellin found that 'previous alcohol, cigarette and marijuana use were each associated with current abuse of prescription opiods in 18-25 year old men, but only marijuana use was associated with subsequent use of prescription opioids in young women'.

NHS Statistics Agency December 2013 showed that more than 20 babies/week are born addicted to drugs, including methadone in England. More than 10,000 newborns had to put into 'cold turkey' at birth. The number with 'neonatal withdrawal symptoms' has risen by 11% in the past 4 years to 1,129 last year.

2013 Varner et al found that smoking pot may double the risk for stillbirth. Cannabis, smoking, illicit drug use and second-hand smoke exposure are linked to an increased risk for stillbirth. 663 stillbirths were enrolled into the study and 1,900 live births. Cannabis increased the odds of stillbirth by more than twice as much a 2.8-fold increase.

2013 Capogrosso et al investigated erectile dysfunction. They found that 1 in 4 men seeking help for newly developing erectile dysfunction (ED) was under 40, nearly half of them having a serious condition. ED is common among older men, the prevalence increases with age. Severe ED was found in 48.8% of younger patients and 40% of the older men. Compared with the older men, younger men had a lower average body mass index, a higher average level of testosterone in the blood and a lower rate of other medical conditions (9.6% cf 41.7%). They had also smoked cigarettes and used illicit drugs. Capogrosso P, Colicchia M, Ventimiglia E, Castagna G, Clementi MC, more frequently than older patients.

2014 Szutorisz et al Found that parental THC exposure leads to compulsive heroin seeking etc in the subsequent generation: electrophysiologically, plasticity was altered at excitatory synapses of the striatal circuitry that is known to mediate compulsive and goal-directed behaviour. These findings demonstate that parental history of germ-Szutorisz H, DiNieriline THC exposure affects the molecular characteristics of the striatum, can impact offspring phenotype, and could possibly confer enhanced risk for psychiatric disorders in the subsequent generation.

2014 Jan Jaques et al in a review of the literature, weeded out the myths of the pregnant woman and her child. Current evidence indicates that cannabis use both during pregnancy and lactation may adversely affect neurodevelopment, especially during periods of critical brain growth both in the developing foetal brain and durinf adolescent maturation, with impacts on neuropsychiatric, behavioural and executive functioning. Future adult productivity and lifetime outcomes may be influenced.

2014 June Pacey et al found that sperm shape and size in young men can be affected by cannabis use. Men who produced ejaculates with less than 4% normal sperm (the current criterium for normal) were nearly twice as likely to have produced a sample in the summer months (June to August) or if they were below 30 or to have used cannabis in the 3 months prior to ejaculation. Alcohol and tobacco had little effect. (Men exposed to paint stripper and lead have similar problems).

The following have endorsed this submission:

- Professor Heather Ashton, Emeritus Professor of Clinical Psychopharmacology, Newcastle University.
- Professor Neil McKeganey, Professor of Drug Misuse Research, University of Glasgow.
- Professor Eric Voth, MD, FACP, Chairman Institute on Global Drug Policy, Editor in chief, The Journal of Global Drug Policy and Practice.
- Dr Ian Oliver, Former Chief Constable of both Central Scotland and Grampian Police, International Consultant on Drugs to the UN, Board member of the International Scientific and Medical Advisory Forum

on Drug Abuse and an elected member of The Institute of Global Drug Policy.

- Dr Michelle Tempest, Liaison Psychiatrist, Addenbrookes Hospital Cambridge.
- Dr Hans-Christian Raabe, GP Manchester. Long-time Campaigner against Cannabis.
- Dr Hans Koeppel MD, Psychiatrist, Swiss Doctors against Drugs. Chair of Scientific Board EURAD (Europe Against drugs).
- Dr Anthony Seldon, Master, Wellington College, Berks.
- Grainne Kenny, International President of EURAD (Europe Against Drugs). Trained Counsellor and Drug Educator.
- Dennis Wrigley, Leader and co-founder, The Maranatha Community, Manchester. (The Maranatha Community has been deeply involved in helping young people with drug problems for over 25 years in many parts of the United Kingdom. Its thousands of members include doctors, scientists, teachers, social workers, counsellors, in addition to numerous voluntary workers).
- Peter O'Loughlin, Director, The Eden Lodge Practice. Drug and Alcohol Recovery Specialist.
- Debra Bell, Founder, Chair, 'Talking About Cannabis'.
- Peter Walker, ex-Headteacher Abbey School, Faversham, Kent. Advisor to the Government on Drug Testing in Schools.
- Dawn Lowe-Watson, Writer, Bereaved Parent.
- Bill Cameron, President Drug-Free Scotland.

....

References

Abel EL, Effects of Prenatal Exposure to Cannabinoids. In Pinkert TM editor, Current Research on the Consequences of Maternal Drug Abuse. National Institute of Drug Abuse: Research Monograph 59. Rockville, MD; US Department of Health and Human Services;1985.

Abel EL, Alcohol Enhancement of Marijuana-Induced Fetotoxicity. Teratology 1985; 31: 35-40.

Astley SJ, Little RE Maternal marijuana use during lactation and infant development at one year. Neurotoxicol Teratol 1990; 12(2): 161-8.

Aversa A, Rossil F, Francomanol D, Bruzzichesl R, Bertonel C, Santiemmal V, Speral G, Early endothelial dysfunction as a marker of vasculogenic erectile dysfunction in young habitual cannabis users. International Journal of Impotence Research 2008, 20, 566-573 doi: 10.1038/ijir.2008.43

Barros M CdeM et al Smoking Marijuana During Pregnancy Alters Newborn Behaviour. Journal of Pediatrics January 2007 119(1).

Berghuis P, Rajnicek AM, Morozov YM, Ross R, Mulder J, Urban GM et al Hardwiring the Brain: Endocannabinoids Shape Neuronal Connectivity. Science 2007 May 25; 316(5828):1212-6.

Blackard C Tennes K Human placental transfer of cannabinoids New England Journal of medicine 1984;311:797.

Bloch E Effects of marijuana and cannabinoids on reproduction, endocrine function, development and chromosomes in KO Fehr and H Kalant (eds) Cannabis and Health hazards. Toronto: Addiction Research Foundation.1983

Bluhm EC, Pollock BH, Olshan AF, *Maternal use of recreational drugs and neuroblastoma in offspring: a report from the Children's Oncology Group (Unitee States).* Cancer Causes Control 2006 Jun: 17(5); 663-9.

Burkman L et al Sperm from Marijuana Smokers Move too Fast too Early, Impairing fertility, UB Research Shows. Annual Meeting Amer Soc of Reprod Med October 13 2003 San Antonio.

Campolongo P, Trezza V, Ratano P, Palmery M, Cuomo V, Developmental consequences of perinatal cannabis exposure: behavioural and neuroendocrine effects in adult rodents. Psychopharmacology DOI 10.1007/s00213-010-1892-x Published online 17th June 2010.

Cates W, Pope JN Gynecomastia and cannabis smoking: A non-association among US army soldiers American journal of Surgery 1977; 134:613-5.

Capogrosso P, Colicchia M, Ventimiglia E, Castagna G, Clementi MC, One Patient out of Four with newly diagnosed Erectile Dysfunction is a Young Man-Worrisome Picture from the Everyday Clinical practice. The Journal of Sexual Medicine 2013: 10: 1833-1841. doi:10.1111/jsm.12179

Copeland KC, Underwood LE, Van Wyk JJ Marijuana smoking and prepubertal arrest Journal of Pediatrics 1980; 96:1079-80.

Cuomo V et al Marijuana use in pregnancy damages children's learning Proceedings of the National Academy of Sciences (DOI: 10.1073/pnas.0537849100) 2003.

Dahl RE A Longitudinal Study of Prenatal Marijuana Use: Effects of Sleep and Arousal at Age Three Years Arch Pediatr Adolesc Med 1995;149:145-50.

Day NL et al Effect of Prenatal Marijuana Exposure on the Cognitive Development of Offspring at Age Three Neurotoxicology and Teratology 1994; 16(2): 169-75.

Day NL, Goldschmidt, Lidush, Thomas, Carrie *Prenatal marijuana exposure contributes to the prediction of marijuana use at age 14*. Addiction Sept 2006; 101(9): 1313-22.

Day NL, Leech SL, Goldschmidt L, *The effects of prenatal marijuana exposure on delinquent behaviours are mediated by measures of neurocognitive functioning*. Neurotoxicol Teratol. 2011 Jan-Feb; 33(1): 129-36.

Dey S et al (Vanderbilt University Medical centre, Nashville) Journal of Clinical Investigation Aug. 2006.

El Marroun et al, Intrauterine *Cabbabis Exposure Affects Fetal Growth Trajectories: The Generation R Study*. J of The American Academy of Child and Adolescent Psychiatry 2010; 48(12) 1173-1181

English DR, Hulse GK, Milne E, Holman CDJ, Bower CI Maternal cannabis use and birth weight: a meta-analysis Addiction Nov 1997; 92(11): page 1553

Fiellin LE, Tetrault JM, Becker WC, Fiellin DA, Hoff RA, Previous use of alcohol, cigarettes and marijuana and subsequent use of prescription opioids in young adults. J Adolesc Health 2013 Feb:52(2): 158-63 Epub 2012 Aug 20.

Fergusson DM, Horwood LJ, Northstone K Maternal use of cannabis and pregnancy outcome BJOG: an International Journal of Obstetrics and Gynaecology 2002; 109:21-7.

Forrester MB, Merz RD, Risk of Selected Birth Defects with Prenatal Illicit Drug Use, Hawaii, 1986-2002. Journal of Toxicology and Environmental Health Part A, Vol 70(1) Dec 2007:7-18.

Frank DA, Rose-Jacobs R, Crooks D, Cabral HJ, Gerteis J, hacker KA, Martin B, Weinstein ZB, Heeren T, Adolescent initiation of licit and illicit substance use: Impact of intrauterine exposures and post-natal exposures to violence. Neurotoxicl. Teratol. 2011 Jan-Feb 33(1): 100-9. Epub. 2010 Jun. 23rd.

Fried PA Marijuana use by pregnant women: Neurobehavioural effects in neonates Drug and Alcohol Dependence 1980;5: 415-24.

Fried PA Marijuana use by pregnant women and effects on offspring: an update. Neurobehavioural Toxicology and Teratology 1982; 4:451-4.

Fried PA, Watkinson B, A Follow-up Study of Attentional Behaviour in Children Exposed Pre-natally to Marijuana, Cigarettes and Alcohol. Neurotoxicology and Teratology 1992; 14: 299-311. .

Fried PA, Watkinson B, Gray R, Differential Effects on Cognitive Functioning in thirteen to sixteen year olds prenatally exposed to cigarettes and marijuana Neurotoxicl Teratol 2003; 25(4): 427-36.

Gibson GT, Baghurst PA, Colley DP, Maternal alcohol, tobacco and cannabis consumption and the outcome of pregnancy Aust and NZ Journal of Obstetrics and Gynecology 1983; 23:15-19.

Goldschmidt L, Day NL, Richardson GA Effects of prenatal marijuana exposure on Child Behaviour at Age Ten Neurotoxicol Teratol 2002; 22(3): 325-36

Goldschmidt L, Richardson G, Willford J, Day N Prenatal Marijuana

Exposure and Intelligence Test Performance at Age 6. Journal of the American Academy of Child and Adolescent Psychiatry 2008; 47(3): 254-263.

Goldschmidt L, Richardson GA, Willford JA, Severtson SG, Day NL, School achievement in 14 year old youths prenatally exposed to marijuana. Neurotoxicol Teratol. 2012 Jan 34(1): 161-7.

Gray KA, Day NL, Leech S, Richardson GA, Prenatal marijuana exposure: effect on child depressive symptoms at ten years of age. Neurotoxicol Teratol. 2005 May-June 27(3); 439-48.

Gray TR, Eiden RD, Leonard KE, Connors GJ, Shisler S, Huestis MA, Identifying Prenatal Cannabis Exposure and Effects of Concurrent Tobacco Exposure on Neonatal Growth Clinical Chemistry 56:9 1442-1450 2010.

Greenland S, Staisch KJ, Brown N, Gross SJ, The effects of marijuana use during pregnancy I. A preliminary epidemiologic study Americal Journal of Obstetrics and Gynaecology 1982a; 143:408-413.

Greenland S, Staisch KJ, Brown N, Gross SJ, Effects of Marijuana on human pregnancy, labour and delivery Neurobehavioral Toxicology and Teratology 1982b; 4:447-450.

Grufferman S, Schwartz AG, Ruymann FB, Mauer HM, Parent's use of cocaine and marijuana and increased risk of rhabdomyosarcoma in their children Cancer, Causes and Control 1993; 4:217-24.

Hall W, Solowij N Lemon J The Health and psychological Consequences of Cannabis Use. Canberra: Australian government Publishing Service; 1994.

Harmon J, Alliapoulios MA, Gynecomastia in marijuana users N Engl J Med 1972; 287: 936.

HaskanyT, Guzman M, Galve-Roperh I, Berghuis P, Devi LA, Mackie K The emerging functions of endocannabinoid signaling during CNS development. Trends in Pharmacological Sciences 2007; 28(2): 88-92.

Hatch EF, Bracken MB Effect of Marijuana Use in Pregnancy on Fetal Growth. Am J of Epidemiology 1986; 24: 986-93.

Hingson R et al Effects of maternal drinking and marijuana use on foetal growth and development Pediatrics 1982; 70:539-46.

Hollister LE Health Aspects of Cannabis Pharmacological reviews 1986;38:1-20.

Huizink AC, Mulder EJ Maternal smoking, drinking or cannabis use during pregnancy and neurobehavioural and cognitive functioning in human offspring Neurosci Biobehav Rev 2006 30(1) 24-41.

Jaques SC, Kingsbury A, Henshcke P, Chomchai C, Clews S, Falconer J, et al, Cannabis, the pregnant woman and her child: weeding out the myths. J. Perinatol. 2014 Jan 23 doi: 10.1038/jp.2013.180 (Epub ahead of print). Institute of Medicine Marijuana and Health Washington DC: National Academy Press; 1982

Keimpema E, Mackie K, Harkany T, Molecular model of cannabis sensitivity in developing neuronal circuits. Pharmacological Sciences volume 32, issue 9, Sep 2011, pages 551-561.

Klonoff-Cohen HS, Natarajan L, Chen RV A prospective study of the effects of female and male marijuana use on in vitro fertilization (IVF) and gamete intrafallopian transfer (GIFT) outcomes Amer J Obst Gynecol 2006; 194:369-76.

Kolodny RC, Masters WH, Kolodner RM, Toro G Depression of plasma testosterone levels after chronic intensive marijuana use New England Journal of Medicine 1974; 290:872-4.

Lacson JCA, Carroll JD, Tuazon E, Castelao EJ, Bernstein L, Cortessis V, Population-based case-control study of recreational drug use and testis cancer risk confirms an association between marijuana use and non-seminoma risk. Cancer 118:5374-5383. doi: 10,1002cncr.27554. 2012

Leavitt J et al Referred to in: Hall W, Solowij N, Lemon J The Health and Psychological Cosequences of Cannabis Use Canberra: Australian Government Publishing Service;994 pages 136-9.

Linn S et al The Association of Marijuana Use with Outcome of Pregnancy Amer J Public Health 1983; 73(10):1161-4.

Lundqvist T Cognitive Dysfunctions in Chronic Cannabis Users Observed

During Treatment: An Integrative Approach Dissertation. Stockholm: Almqvist and Wiksell International; 1995.

Mendelson JH, Mello NK, Effects of marijuana on neuroendocrine hormones in human males and females In M Braude and JP Ludford (eds) Marijuana Effects on the Endocrine and Reproductive Systems Rockville Maryland: National Institute on Drug Abuse.1984.

Marroun HE, Hudziak JJ, Tiemeler H, Creemers H, Steegers EA, Jaddoe VW, Hofman A, Verhulst FC, van den Brink W, Hulzink AC, Intrauterine cannabis exposure leads to more aggressive behaviour and attention problems in 18-month old girls. Drug Alcohol Dependece 2011 Apr4 (Epub ahead of publication)

Nahas GG Toxicology and Pharmacology In GG Nahas Marijuana in Science and Medicine: New York Raven Press.1984.

Nahas GG, Frick H Developmental effects of cannabis Neurotoxicology 1987; 7:381-95. National Academy of Sciences 82

Nahas GG, Sutin KM, Harvey DJ, Agurell S, eds Marijuana and Medicine 1999 Humana Press Totowa, NJ.

Nahas GG, Frick HC, Lattimer JK, Latour C, Harvey D, Pharmakinetics of THC in brain and testes, male gametotoxicity and premature apoptosis of spermatozoa. Hum Psychopharmacol. 2002 Mar; 17(2): 103-113.

Neglia JP, Buckley JD, Robinson LL Maternal marijuana use and leukaemia in offspring In GG Nahas and C Latour (eds) Physiology of Illicit Drugs: Cannabis, Cocaine, Opiates. Oxford Pergamon Press. 1991.

NHS Statistics Agency, following report by the CSJ, and a PQ answered by Dr Dan Poulter, Health Minister. Dec 2013

Pacey A, Povey A, Clyma J, Mcnamee R, Moore H, Baillie, Cherry N, Modifiable and non-modifiable risk factors for poor sperm morphology. Human Reproduction, June 2014, DOI: 10.1093/humrep/deu 116.

Paria BC, Song H, Wang X, Schmid PC, Krebsbach RJ, Schmid HHO, Bonner TI, Zimmer A, Dey SK *Dysregulated Cannabinoid Signalling Disrupts Uterine Receptivity for Embryo Implantation* J Biol Chem 2001; 276(23): 20523-28.

Psychoyos D, Vinod YK, (2012) Marijuana, *Spice* 'herbal high', and early neural development: implications for rescheduling and legalization Drug Test Analysis. Doi:10.1002/dta.1390 August 2012

Richardson GA, Ryan C, Willford J, Day NL, Goldscmidt L, Prenatal alcohol and marijuana exposure: effects on neuropsychological outcomes at 10 years. Neurotoxicol Teratol. 2002 May-June 24(3): 309-20.

Robison LI, Buckley JD, Daigle AE, Wells R Benjamin D Arthur D, Hammond GD Maternal drug use and the risk of childhood non-lymphoblastic leukaemia among offspring: An epidemiological investigation implicating marijuana Cancer 1989; 63:1904-11.

Rosencrantz H Cannabis components and responses of neuroendochrine-reproductive targets: an Overview In DJ Harvey, W Paton and GG Nahas (eds) Marijuana '84: Proceedings of the Oxford Symposium on Cannabis Oxford IRL Press 1985.

Schuel H, Burkman LJ, Lippes J, Crickard K, Mahony MC, Giuffrida A, Picone RP, Makriyannis A, Evidence that anandamide-signaling regulates human sperm functions required for fertilization. Mol Reprod Dev 2002; 63(3):376-87.

Scragg RK, Mitchell EA, Ford RP, Thompson JM, Taylor BJ, Stewart AW Maternal cannabis use in sudden death syndrome Acta Paediatr 2001; 90(1): 57-60.

Shamloul R, Bella AJ, Impact of Cannabis Use on Male Sexual Health. The Journal of Sexual Medicine, 2001 January 26th.

Sherwood RA, Keating J, Kavvadia V, Greenough A, Peters TJ Substance misuse in early pregnancy and relationship to fetal outcome European Journal Paediatrics 1999; 158 (6): 488-92.

Shiono PH, Klebanoff MA, Nugent RP et al The impact of cocaine and marijuana use on low birth weight and preterm birth: a multicenter study Am J Obstet Gynecol 1995; 172:19-27.

Szutorisz H, DiNieri JA, Sweet E, Egervari G, Michaelides M, Carter, JM, Ren Y, Miller ML, Blitzer RD, Hurd Y, Parental THC Exposure Leads to Compulsive Heroin-seeking and altered Striatal Synaptic Plasticity, in the Subsequent Generation. Neuropsychopharmacology doi: 10.1038/npp.2013.352. January 2014.

Tennes K et al Marijuana: prenatal and postnatal exposure in the human In TM Pinkert (ed) Current Research on the Consequences of Maternal Drug Abuse National institute on drug Abuse Research monograph No. 59 Rockville MD: US Department of Health and Human services. 1985.

Varner M, Reddy U, Rabin MD, Walter R, Study: Using Tobacco, drugs in pregnancy can double stillbirth risk January 2014 *Obstetrics & Gynecology*

Viagra Sunday Mail 19th May 2008 Doctors blame cannabis for rise in NHS spending on Viagra.

Wang H, Matsumoto H, Guo Y, Paria BC, Roberts RL, Key SK *Differential G protein-coupling cannabinoid receptor signaling by anandamide directs blastocyst activation for implantation* PNAS (Proceedings of the National Academy of Sciences of The United States of America) 2003; 100(25) 14914-19.

Wenger T, Croix D, Tramu G, Leonardeli J, Effects of delta-9-tetrahydrocannabinol on pregnancy, puberty and the neuroendocrine system In L Murphy and A Bartke (eds) Marijuana/Cannabinoids: Neurobiology and Neurophysiology Boca Raton: CRC Press. 1992.

Willford JA, Chandler LS, Goldschmidt L, Day NL, Effects of pre-natal tobacco, alcohol and marijuana exposure on processing speed, visual-motor coordination, and interhemispheric transfer. Neurotoxicol. Teratol. 2010 Nov-Dec 32(6):580-8.

Zuckerman B et al Effects of maternal marijuana and cocaine use on fetal growth. New England Journal of Medicine 1989; 320:762-8.

Zhu W, Friedman H, Klein T Delta 9 Tetrahydrocannabinol Induces Apoptosis in Macrophages and Lymphocytes: Involvement of Bcl-2 and Caspase-1 J of Pharmacology and Experimental Therapeutics 1998; 286(2): 1103-9.

Mary Brett is a retired biology teacher. She taught in a mixed comprehensive school in Glasgow for 5 years, then in an English Grammar school (selective) for boys for over 30 years where she was in charge of Health Education.

She has campaigned against cannabis for well over 20 years and is now Chair of the drug prevention charity, CanSS (Cannabis Skunk Sense, www.cannabisskunksense.co.uk. CanSS provides the admin for the APPG (All Party Parliamentary Group) on Cannabis and Children in the United Kingdom's House of Commons. She is also a member of WFAD (World Forum Against Drugs) and an ex-Vice President of Eurad.

**MOURAD W. GABRIEL, GRETA M. WENGERT,
J. MARK HIGLEY, SHANE KROGAN,
WARREN SARGENT, DEANA L. CLIFFORD**
Integral Ecology Research Center,
Blue Lake, California

Silent Forests?
Rodenticides on Illegal Marijuana Crops Harm Wildlife

THE FISHER (MARTES PENNANTI) is a cat-sized carnivore found in coniferous and mixed conifer and hardwood forests across Canada and in four regions of the United States, including New England, the Great Lakes, the northern Rockies, and the Pacific Northwest. Now a candidate species for listing under the Endangered Species Act, fishers in California are falling victim to rodenticides used on illegal marijuana crops scattered throughout the state's public and tribal lands. (Credit: John Jacobson/Washington Department of Fish and Wildlife)

Another mortality signal on the radio collar of a fisher (Martes pennanti) pulses on a wet spring morning, and fear of a repeat of the previous spring's mortalities looms in the backs of our minds. Hoopa tribal biologists scramble to recover the fisher quickly so that a necropsy can be performed to determine cause of death. The field crew reports back that the fisher is not dead but lethargic and lurching on the ground when it attempts to seek cover from approaching biologists. A conference call among researchers, a wildlife pathologist, and a veterinary toxicologist follows to determine the next course of action. Unfortunately, the consensus is humane euthanization. Though testing is ongoing, this is likely the sixth monitored fisher in California that has died from second-generation anticoagulant rodenticide (SGAR) toxicosis since 2009.

Linking SGARs to multiple deaths of a rare forest carnivore has been an alarming discovery. Even more unsettling: We've learned that these deaths appear to be linked to illegal marijuana cultivation on community and public lands — a finding that raises serious concerns for the health of many species of wildlife including fishers, an Endangered Species Act candidate.

A Growing Concern

Beginning in 2008, full necropsies including toxicological screens—done at the University of California-Davis School of Veterinary Medicine and the California Animal Health and Food Safety Laboratory (CAHFS)—have been conducted to determine proximate and ultimate causes of mortality for fishers from the Hoopa Valley Reservation Fisher Project (HVRFP), Sierra Nevada Adaptive Management Project (SNAMP), and the U.S. Forest Service (USFS) Kings River Fisher Project (KRFP). These ongoing, long-term demographic projects encompass both tribal community forests within the

HVRFP and public lands including Yosemite National Park and Sierra National Forest in the SNAMP and KRFP study areas.

Toxicology screening of 58 fishers from these community and public lands revealed that nearly 80 percent of the fishers had been exposed to anticoagulant rodenticide (AR) poisons, with 96 percent of those exposures being SGARs – results that we published recently in PLoS ONE (Gabriel et al. 2012). Concerned about this trend, we led an interdisciplinary collaboration including multiple stakeholders from the Hoopa Tribe, Integral Ecology Research Center, USFS, U.S. Fish and Wildlife Service, CAHFS, UC-Davis, SNAMP, and California Department of Fish and Wildlife, pooling together resources and expertise for a comprehensive approach to evaluate this emerging threat.

Spatial modeling suggested that fishers were exposed to SGARs ubiquitously throughout the study areas, contradicting current thought that wildlife are at greatest risk to these toxicants near agricultural, urban, or peri-urban settings, where the pesticides are legally used to eradicate or suppress rodent pest populations. However, lifetime monitoring of the California fishers showed that most of the exposed or poisoned individuals never overlapped any of those land-use types. In addition, the use of SGARs within the study areas, in adjacent timberlands, or within campgrounds would violate current state and federal regulations. As a result, our suspicions gravitated towards undiscovered illicit uses throughout the project areas. These suspicions were essentially confirmed after federal, state, and local law enforcement officers verified that the poisons were present at most marijuana cultivation sites found on public and tribal lands.

All of our documented SGAR fisher mortalities occurred from late April through early June, which is prime-time for marijuana seedling planting in California and likely the period of heaviest toxicant use to protect young plants from rodent damage. Regrettably, this is also a key time for female fishers to rear their kits. That unfortunate timing materialized when we discovered a lactating female fisher dead from SGAR poisoning in the Southern Sierra Nevadas. (California currently has two isolated native fisher populations, one within the northwestern coastal mountains, where population estimates are unknown, and another within the Southern Sierra Nevadas, where estimates suggest fewer than 300 adults [Spencer et al. 2011]). Presumably, the dead mother's kits also died due to den abandonment.

In a separate instance, a rescue attempt on an abandoned fisher kit still dependent on its mother's milk was unsuccessful, and the kit was found dead of starvation. Most disconcerting was that SGARs were detected in the kit's tissues. This unexpected finding verified a transplacental or milk transfer of a SGAR from mother to kit, raising concern about fetotoxic or bioaccumulation effects of these pesticides, which are currently unknown.

These findings underscore the need to understand not only the direct impacts of these toxicants, but other possible indirect impacts that fishers and other wildlife may face at the population level. For example, we detected an average of 1.6 different types of ARs per fisher, with some fishers testing positive for four different toxic compounds. There are no data on the possible interactions of two, three, or even four different ARs, or the effects they might have on animal health. Furthermore, we cannot yet determine whether a threshold level of exposure exists beyond which an animal cannot recover, since some fishers died with low levels of SGARs while others displayed no clinical signs even withmuch higher exposures. We wonder if these toxicants at sub-lethal doses lower resistance to environmental stressors, as seen in other studies, and whether the distribution of SGARs within the landscape will limit prey availability and create sink habitats near cultivation sites. This is just the beginning of a long list of potential cascading impacts now being discussed in California.

Dots scattered through California's Sierra and Sequoia National Forests represent some 600 illegal marijuana grow sites reclaimed by crews who removed trash, hazardous chemicals, water diversions, and rudimentary shelters left by growers. Blue shading represents current range of the fisher within the southern Sierra Nevadas, where the population is estimated at fewer than 300 adults. (Credit: Greta M. Wengert)

Problem Spreading Like Weeds

Illegal marijuana growing is not just a problem for wildlife. The High Sierra Volunteer Trail Crew is a nonprofit trail-maintenance crew that has spent the past seven years maintaining and cleaning trails throughout the Sierra Nevadas' national forests. In the mid-2000s, the group realized that risks associated with large-scale marijuana production throughout most, if not all, California national forests threatened backcountry use of public lands. Since then, the trail crew's Environmental Reclamation Team (ERT) has remediated more than 600 large-scale marijuana cultivation sites on public lands. The numbers are daunting, especially when considering that these 600 sites were in only two of California's 17 national forests and may constitute only a fraction of the actual marijuana cultivation sites that exist in these forests. Tommy Lanier, Director of the National Marijuana Initiative, a White House supported program, states that "60 percent to 70 percent of the national marijuana seizures come from California annually, and of those totals, about 60 percent comes from public lands."

Based on data from ERT-remediated sites, at least 50 percent of them have SGARs. Beyond finding anticoagulant rodenticides, the team and other remediation groups frequently find and remove restricted and banned pesticides including organo phosphates, organochlorines, and carbamates as well as thousands of pounds of nitrogen-rich fertilizers. Many of the discovered pesticides have been banned for use in the U.S., Canada, and the European Union, specifically certain carbamates, which gained notoriety worldwide after an explosion of public awareness about their use to kill African wildlife. Unfortunately, these same malicious uses are occurring in California, where marijuana cultivators place pourable carbamate pesticides in opened tuna or sardine cans in order to kill black bears, gray foxes, raccoons, and other carnivores that damage marijuana plants or raid food caches at grow-site encampments.

In many cases, law enforcement officers approaching grow sites observe wildlife exposed to what officers call "wildlife bombs" due to their high potential for mass wildlife killing. For example, as federal and state officers approached a grow site in Northern California, they discovered a black bear and her cubs seizing and convulsing as they slowly succumbed to the neurological effects of these pesticides. Because toxicants are usually dispersed throughout cultivation sites, it is remarkably difficult to detect and remove all pesticide threats.

Funding to document, quantify, and remediate the damage caused by illegal marijuana cultivation on public and tribal lands has been difficult to secure through state or federal agencies or even private foundations, possibly due to the common misperceptions that illegal marijuana cultivation is not an environmental but rather a social issue, and that it is not a significant threat to wildlife. Yet we propose that funding is strongly warranted to help researchers investigate toxicant exposure and implications throughout the forests' trophic levels, and to study impacts on all species of conservation concern, including fishers and the northern spotted owl.

Another common misperception is that it is the responsibility of law enforcement to not only protect our natural resources at illegal marijuana sites, but also to remove pesticides and remediate the sites. In truth, there is currently no standardized system for grow-site remediation. Recently, for example, we encountered more than 10 pounds of SGARs and 20 pounds of metaldehyde and carbamates from a single site that law enforcement officers had dismantled within fisher and northern spotted owl territories. Most of these toxicants were left untouched out of concern for the safety of the officers, who are not trained to handle and transport these highly toxic chemicals, especially in the frequent situation where these chemicals are unlabeled. Accordingly, without documentation of the environmental damage and threats from toxicants, and without funding for properly trained personnel, most poisons will continue to be left at grow sites, where they remain a catastrophic threat to wildlife.

Effects Extend beyond Poison

Environmental threats from large-scale marijuana cultivation are certainly not limited to toxicant contamination. At most grow sites, it is standard practice to clear patches of forest within riparian corridors in order to provide enough sunlight for growing plants. The cumulative impact of these practices across the California landscape is unknown, but disheartening in its potential. Last year, at a site within the Hoopa Valley Indian Reservation in northern California, where 26,600 marijuana plants were removed, several acres of hardwood-conifer and alder forest had been cleared along one of the most productive Chinook and Coho salmon-bearing streams in the area. Under no circumstance would this clearing be allowed under the Tribe's management plans or current state or federal regulations established to protect habitat for the salmon.

Because growers prefer areas with a constant and abundant water supply, it is these sensitive habitats that suffer the greatest impacts from marijuana cultivation. Water diversions and pesticide-filled cisterns within streambeds feeding miles of plastic irrigation lines are all-too-familiar a sight. Human waste throughout these sites is also widespread, and because many of the sites on public and tribal lands are inhabited for several months of the year by drug-traffic organizations, extensive camp systems are set up with associated trash dumps and human latrine sites just meters away from water sources.

The camps and plantations are often guarded by armed drug traffickers, so concern for the safety of field crews, students, and biologists working on these lands is ever pressing. Wildlife professionals are fearful of unwittingly running into armed growers at active grow sites, with good reason. Recently, a federal biologist in the southern Sierra Nevadas was chased by armed growers for 40 minutes through the national forest. "When we lost radio contact at one point for 10 minutes, we feared that the biologist was captured or possibly dead," says project supervisor Jodi Tucker of Sequoia National Forest. In another incident in the 2012 field season, biologists surveying for northern spotted owls on the Hoopa Reservation were shot at by suspected illegal growers with high-caliber assault rifles. Luckily, no one was injured, but biologists avoided the survey area until the threat was addressed.

Due to heighted safety concerns and emerging patterns like these over the past several years, wildlife crews now are often composed of two individuals, whereas before, biologists worked independently in the field. The effects of these changes have not been fully ascertained, but it can be assumed that increased labor costs coupled with increased equipment and vehicle expenditures are affecting the size, duration, and thoroughness of data for many studies on California's public and tribal lands.

Because wildlife biologists are also avoiding some study areas due to safety concerns, study designs are now being altered to avoid known grow sites, thus further impacting quality and completeness of data. Research ecologist Craig Thompson from the USFS Pacific Southwest Research Station estimates that during each field season, 10 to 25 percent of the Kings River Fisher Project area becomes inaccessible due to safety concerns. In another telling example during the 2010-2011 field season, two radio-collared fishers in this study area pulsed mortality signals but could not be recovered due to their locations near known grow sites. Eventually, under escort by armed law enforcement officers, biologists recovered the collars, yet the carcasses — and any evidence of cause of death or rodenticide toxicosis — were long destroyed.

In his *Science* editorial "The Tragedy of the Commons," Garret Hardin lamented the loss of our public resources due to the greed and inconsid eration of some individuals (Hardin 1968). We believe the vast and ever-growing misuse of our public and tribal forests for the financial benefit of a few individuals is an enormous threat to these resources and a deplorable tragedy of the commons. Our public and tribal land and agencies are being hit on two fronts: first by having to endure the illegal use, take, and destruction of natural resources without our permission, then having to support the financial burden of renewing these lands from the disastrous ecosystem degradation that illicit cultivation produces. Regrettably, most of this is occurring without the knowledge of the public, whose land it is. Though this is a sad story that often brings surprise, disgust, and a feeling of helplessness in those hearing it for the first time, in the words of Rachel Carson, "The public must decide whether it wishes to continue on the present road, and it can do so only when in full possession of the facts."

Reprinted with permission. *Wildlife Society News*. Spring 2013, April 11, 2013.

Marijuana Cultivation

Marijuana cultivation, whether trespass grows on public or tribal lands or the cultivation on private lands, has significant impacts on California's natural resources. These ecological impacts run deep and wide in many ways and add more burden to the state's currently strained natural resources. Impacts range from the malicious poisoning of Federally and State-listed wildlife species with banned and restricted-use pesticides, poaching of game, illegal water diversions, habitat destruction, and the contamination of water and soil. Furthermore, illegal marijuana cultivation impacts the safety of natural resource professionals in the field and deters young professionals from working in our state. These safety risks have come to fruition in the form of physical intimidation, shootings, and the murder of a forester. In addition, illegal marijuana cultivation has desecrated culturally and spiritually significant tribal lands as well as endangered the health of law enforcement and the public from the indiscriminate use of hazardous chemicals. Illegal marijuana cultivation has also cost Californians fiscally. Wildland fire suppression directly attributed to trespass marijuana cultivation in California cost the public $55 million (110,235 acres burned). Publically funded research and conservation projects incur hundreds of thousands of dollars in additional costs due to safety concerns each year. Due to the complexity of the effects of this activity, an interdisciplinary approach has been initiated in order to generate an understanding of the current threats, address the impacts, and advise natural resource managers and policy-makers towards potential solutions. In turn, the information generated from investigating these impacts can provide a foundation for education of the public to become engaged and involved in developing solutions.

Dr.Mourad Gabriel

Dr. Mourad Gabriel is an ecologist whose research focuses on investigating and understanding threats to wildlife populations of conservation concern from both infectious and non-infectious disease agents. His current research concentrated on the vast environmental impacts marijuana cultivation has on California's natural resources. He completed both his Bachelor's and Master's degrees at Humboldt State University and his Doctorate in Comparative Pathology at the University of California Davis, School of Veterinary Medicine. He is the executive director of Integral Ecology Research Center, a non-profit scientific research organization headquartered in Northwestern California, which leads several interdisciplinary national and international research projects. Dr. Gabriel has authored numerous ecological scientific publications and book chapters and mentored students working on conservation projects in both the field and laboratory. He resides in Northwestern California where he, his wife and daughter, try to spend as much time as possible outdoors enjoying our public lands.Greta M. Wengert is a Wildlife Ecologist with the Integral Ecology Research Center.

J. Mark Higley is a Wildlife Biologist with Hoopa Tribal Forestry.

Shane Krogan is Executive Director of the High Sierra Volunteer Trail Crew.

Warren Sargent is a Forensic Engineer with the High Sierra Volunteer Trail Crew.

Deana L. Clifford, DVM, Ph.D., is a Wildlife Veterinarian with the California Department of Fish and Wildlife.

MARA W. STEWART
University of Wisconsin School of Medicine and Public Health, Dept. of Pediatrics

MEGAN A. MORENO, MD, MPH, MSEd
Center for Child Health Behavior and Development, Seattle, WA

Changes in Attitudes, Intentions, and Behaviors toward Tobacco and Marijuana during US Students' First Year of College

Abstract

Tobacco and marijuana are commonly used by college students and have negative health effects. The purpose of this study was to understand how students' attitudes, intentions, and behaviors toward tobacco and marijuana change during freshman year and to examine how attitude and intention predict use of these substances. 275 college students completed phone interviews before and after their freshman year. The identical interviews assessed students' attitudes, intentions, and behaviors toward both substances. Attitudes and intentions increased significantly. 12.2% of participants initiated tobacco use and 13.5% initiated marijuana use. Only intention predicted tobacco initiation, while both attitude and intention predicted marijuana initiation. Overall, attitudes, intentions, and behaviors changed significantly toward favored use.

Predictors of use varied by substance, suggesting that different prevention approaches may be beneficial

Introduction

The transition from high school to college is marked by newfound independence, intellectual growth, and repeated encounters with substance use and abuse. Tobacco and marijuana are among the most abused substances by university students in the United States.[1] While cigarette smoking among adolescents is currently at a historic low,[2] marijuana use continues to increase.[3] Recent data from the National College Health Assessment shows that roughly one-third of all college students have tried either a hookah with tobacco or cigarettes, and over 37% have tried marijuana.[4] Given that 80% to 90% of tobacco smokers begin smoking during adolescence or early adulthood and roughly 25% of marijuana consumers initiate use after starting college,[5,6] first-year college students comprise a vital target group for tobacco and marijuana intervention.

Tobacco use consequences and patterns

Tobacco use during the college years can lead to physical, mental, and emotional harm as well as addiction. As the leading preventable cause of death in the United States, tobacco use is linked to an array of human cancers, cardiovascular diseases, and respiratory diseases.[7] Among students who are daily tobacco users, nicotine use has been associated with poorer working memory performance and neurotoxicity.[8] Furthermore, cessation of tobacco use has been associated with withdrawal symptoms including depression, anxiety, nicotine cravings, and disruption of memory.[8] Although cigarettes account for much of college students' tobacco use, it is also understood that most students who have used tobacco have used more than one method of consumption.[9]

Despite its adverse health effects, tobacco use has become an integral part of the college experience. Among U.S. college students, over half of current smokers are social smokers, meaning they smoke primarily with others.[10] When compared to the general adult population, young adult smokers are less likely to smoke every day and they consume fewer cigarettes on a daily basis.[10] However, social smoking during adolescence has the potential to lead to life-long addiction. Social smokers represent a unique subset of tobacco users because they generally believe that they are not addicted to nicotine and will not continue to smoke after leaving the college environment.[10] Research contradicts these assumptions, showing that adolescents who smoke only a few cigarettes per month and those who have smoked as few as 100 cigarettes total can suffer physical and psychological withdrawal symptoms when they attempt to quit using tobacco and are deprived of nicotine.[6] The tobacco industry has long recognized the importance of social influence on smoking and employs marketing strategies that target young adults across bars, clubs, and college campuses.[9] Because college freshmen attempt to define themselves socially during their transition to college,[11] they may be especially susceptible to the influence of peers and of the tobacco industry.

Despite strategic marketing ploys by the tobacco industry, patterns of tobacco use among college students during the past 15 years have shown a marked decrease in current (past-30-day) use. In 1999, 31% of U.S. college students had smoked within the past month and in 2011 only 15% had smoked within the past month.[12] A comparison of tobacco use across different class standings demonstrated an upward trajectory of tobacco use during the college years, showing that more college seniors use cigarettes and smokeless tobacco products than do freshmen.[13] Thus, although overall tobacco use is currently at historic lows, a student's freshman year may be a critical time in which he or she establishes later-college and potentially life-long use.

Marijuana use consequences and patterns

As the relationship between college students and their tobacco use becomes more clearly understood, a growing body of research is also revealing a relationship between college students and marijuana use. Marijuana is the most prevalent illicit drug used by adolescents and young adults.[5] Although recent data suggests that marijuana is less damaging to lungs than tobacco,[14] long-term marijuana use has been associated with other adverse physical health outcomes including respiratory disorders, injury to airway tissue, and impaired immune function.[15,16] Furthermore, marijuana use has been associated with neuropsychological and cognitive decline from childhood to midlife, even after adjusting for years of education, and has also been associated with the development of certain features of schizophrenia.[3,17]

While data exists on the long-term physical and psychological effects of marijuana, there is also increasing evidence suggesting marijuana impacts a student's social transition to college. At the time of matriculation, first-year students significantly misperceive campus norms for marijuana use, estimating that almost every student has used in the last 30 days.[18] Additionally, 40.5% of entering students perceive the campus atmosphere to be one that promotes marijuana use.[18] A related study found that 74% of students who did not use marijuana prior to college were offered marijuana during college and, of those individuals, 54% initiated marijuana use.[5] Many factors appear to contribute to increased marijuana use during this transition, including decreased adult supervision, overall greater personal freedom, increased availability and opportunity, and a sense of perceived anonymity in the college community.[19]

The trajectory of marijuana use among college students in the past 20 years shows an overall upward trend. From 1991 through 1998, annual and daily prevalence of marijuana use increased significantly among the college population and, after a period of decline in the early part of the millennium, both annual and daily marijuana use again increased.[12] By 2011, about one-third of college students had used marijuana in the past year and 19.4% were current (past-30-day) users.[12] Data shows that marijuana use continues to increase during the college years, with more college seniors using marijuana than freshmen.[13] Therefore, freshman year may be the most beneficial time for marijuana interventions.

Motivations for tobacco and marijuana use

Although both tobacco and marijuana are known to produce negative physical consequences, trends in regulation of each are largely dissimilar. Over the past few decades, billions of dollars have been poured into anti-tobacco media campaigns.[20] Furthermore, almost every state and the federal government have increased tobacco taxes in recent years in an effort to reduce tobacco use and generate revenue.[21] Concurrently, 18 states and Washington, D.C. have passed laws sanctioning medical marijuana use and, in the November 2012 election cycle, two of these states passed additional legislation legalizing recreational marijuana use. Although little empirical evidence exists on this matter, the opposing treatment of tobacco and marijuana by society may lead young adults to develop different sets of beliefs about these substances.

While much is known about college students' substance use behaviors, the adverse effects of these substances, and the political debate surrounding them, little is known about what prompts students to use tobacco and marijuana during their transition to college. The Theory of Planned Behavior has been used successfully as a theoretical framework in numerous adolescent substance use studies.[22,23] The theory suggests that a person's behavior is determined by his or her intentions to perform the behavior. This intention, in turn, is a function of his or her attitudes toward the behavior.[24] Therefore, understanding students' attitudes and intentions is the first step in predicting substance use behaviors and developing interventions. It is unknown, however, whether there is stability or change in the attitudes and intentions that affect behaviors toward tobacco and marijuana in the transition from high school to college. By understanding these factors and how they interrelate, interventions that specifically target each substance can be developed. The purpose of this study was threefold: (1) to understand how students' attitudes, intentions, and behaviors toward tobacco and marijuana change during their first year of college, (2) to understand how students' methods of consumption of these substances change during their first year, and (3) to examine how attitude and intention predict initiation or maintained use of these substances.

Methods

Data for this study was collected between May 15, 2011 and August 5, 2012 and received approval from the Institutional Review Boards of the University of Wisconsin – Madison and the Seattle Children's Research Institute.

Setting and Recruitment

Recruitment efforts began after receiving institutional review board approval from the relevant institutions. Incoming college freshmen from the University of Wisconsin—Madison and the University of Washington – Seattle were recruited for a longitudinal study about health behaviors among college students. These large, state universities were selected based on structural similarity and geographical separation. The separation allowed for differences in overall student culture, which likely led to increased heterogeneity in the sample.

Students were eligible if they were between the ages of 17 and 19 years and enrolled as freshmen for Fall 2011 at one of the two study universities. Participants were randomly selected from freshman rosters, which were provided by the universities upon receiving IRB approval. After generating a list of potential participants, students were recruited via an initial announcement postcard and then received up to three rounds of emails and phone calls. The study design included a pre-college baseline assessment, which required that students' first interviews occurred before they arrived on campus. Consequently, students who were already on campus for early-enrollment programs were excluded from participation. Participants ages 18 and older provided oral consent before their first telephone interview. In cases where the student was a minor, oral consent was required from both a parent and the participant.

Procedure

Telephone interviews were conducted by trained research assistants at two different time periods. Baseline interviews were completed between June and September 2011 (Time 1) before students arrived at their respective schools. Follow-up interviews were conducted between May and August 2012 after the students' first year of college was complete (Time 2). Participants were contacted by a member of the research team when it was time to schedule an interview and were given a choice of time slots based on mutual availability. The identical interviews assessed students' attitudes, intentions, and behaviors toward tobacco and marijuana based on a series of self-report scales. Participants received incentive payments of $25 for completing the first interview and $30 for completing the second interview. Interview responses were entered into a database, quality checked for entering errors by a different research assistant, and compiled for data analysis at the conclusion of the study. Telephone interviews were used for this study because many participants were more than an hour away from the primary research site, and because phone interviews have been used successfully in the past as a way to interview participants regarding stigmatizing topics such as risky health behaviors.[25,26] In order to further minimize the influence of the social desirability bias, interviewers avoided the use of leading questions and emphasized the strict confidentiality of the study at several points throughout the interview.

Measurements

In accordance with the Theory of Planned Behavior, the interviews assessed students' attitudes, intentions, and behaviors regarding tobacco and marijuana through the use of several validated self-report measures. Demographic information including gender, university, type of housing, and ethnicity was also obtained at Time 1.

Attitudes

Attitudes toward both substances were measured with the question, "On a scale between 0 and 6, with 0 as very negative, 3 as neutral, and 6 as very positive, what would you say your own attitude towards (tobacco, marijuana) is?" This question was developed based on previous work that utilized Likert scales to assess young adults' attitudes towards alcohol. [27-29] The current study modified this approach to assess attitudes toward tobacco and marijuana. Participants' responses to this question were scored and categorized exactly as they appeared on the Likert scale, with 0 = very negative, 1 = negative, 2 = somewhat negative, 3 = neutral/don't know, 4 = somewhat positive, 5 = positive, and 6 = very positive.

Intentions

If participants had never used the substance in question, or were not current (past-28-day) users, they were asked, "How likely do you think it is that you will consume this substance in the next 6 months? Please answer from 0 'not at all likely' to 5 'very likely.'" This scale has been used for alcohol assessment in previous work and was found to have an alpha of 0.93.[27] The current study modified this approach to assess tobacco and marijuana intentions. Participants' responses to this question were scored and categorized exactly as they appeared on the Likert scale, with 0 = not at all likely, 1 = unlikely, 2 = somewhat unlikely, 3 = somewhat likely, 4 = likely, and 5 = very likely.

Behaviors

Lifetime use was measured with the question, "Have you ever used (tobacco, marijuana) in your life?" If a participant had ever used tobacco or marijuana, the interviewer read a list of possible methods by which the substance may have been consumed. Participants were instructed to say yes or no to each method and were then asked if there were any other methods by which they had consumed the substance. Students were also asked how old they were when they first tried (tobacco, marijuana) and whether they had used it in the past 28 days.

Data Analysis

Descriptive statistics were calculated. The first purpose of the study was to understand how students' attitudes, intentions, and behaviors towards tobacco and marijuana use change during their first year of college. Because data was not normally distributed, Wilcoxon signed-rank tests for paired data were used to assess these changes between Time 1 and Time 2.

Another purpose of the study was to examine how attitude and intention predict initiation or maintained use of these substances. To understand these relationships, categories of participants' substance use were first defined. The four categories included (1) Tobacco Initiators, who had never used tobacco at Time 1 but had used it by Time 2, (2) Tobacco Maintainers, who had used tobacco at Time 1 and were current users at Time 2, (3) Marijuana Initiators had never used marijuana at Time 1 but had used it by Time 2, and (4) Marijuana Maintainers, who had used marijuana at Time 1 and were current users at Time 2.

For each category, logistic regression models were used

to assess predictors of tobacco or marijuana use at Time 2. Logistic regression models were chosen so that odds ratios could be used to compare the relative odds of the occurrence of the outcome of interest given exposure to the variable of interest and to compare the magnitude of these predictor variables as risk factors for that outcome.

Model 1 assessed predictors of initiation of tobacco use at Time 2. In this model, only participants who reported no lifetime tobacco use at Time 1 were included. Lifetime use of tobacco at Time 2 was the outcome or dependent variable. Predictor or independent variables included attitude towards tobacco and intention to use tobacco reported at Time 1. Model 2 assessed ongoing or maintained tobacco use. In this model, only participants who reported lifetime tobacco use at Time 1 were included. Predictor or independent variables included attitude towards and intention to use tobacco reported at Time 1.

Similarly, Model 3 assessed predictors of marijuana initiation at Time 2. In this model, only participants who reported no lifetime marijuana use at Time 1 were included. Lifetime use of marijuana was the outcome or dependent variable. Predictor or independent variables included attitude towards marijuana and intention to use marijuana reported at Time 1. Model 4 assessed ongoing or maintained marijuana use. In this model, participants who reported lifetime marijuana use at Time 1 were included. Predictor or independent variables included attitude towards and intention to use marijuana reported at Time 1. All models were adjusted for gender and ethnicity. Because of small numbers of some ethnic groups, in all analyses ethnicity was categorized as white or non-white.

All *P* values were 2-sided, and $P < 0.05$ was used to indicate statistical significance. Statistical analyses were performed using Stata version 10 (StataCorp: College Station, TX).

Results

Overall, there was a 52.8% participation rate; 275 participants completed both interviews (81.4%). Among participants, 59.3% attended the University of Wisconsin–Madison and 40.7% attended the University of Washington Seattle. Participants were 57.1% female. The majority of participants (74.9%) were Caucasian; 11.6% were Asian, 3.3% were Hispanic, 1.5% were African American/black, 6.9% were more than one ethnicity, and 1.8% were a different ethnicity. The majority of students (82.9%) lived in a school dormitory, 9.4% lived in a fraternity or sorority, 3.3% lived with a parent or guardian, and 4.4% had a different living arrangement. Both universities have a slightly higher ratio of females to males and predominantly Caucasian student bodies, which is consistent with the demographics of this study. Table 1 summarizes demographic data.

TABLE 1

Demographic Information for First-Year College Student Participants		
N=275	**N**	**%**
Gender		
Male	118	42.9
Female	157	57.1
University		
University of Wisconsin, Madison	163	59.3
University of Washington, Seattle	112	40.7
Ethnicity		
Caucasian/white	206	74.9
Asian	32	11.6
Hispanic	9	3.3
African American/black	4	1.5
More than One	19	6.9
Other	5	1.8
Housing		
School Dormitory	228	82.9
Fraternity/Sorority	26	9.4
Parent's House	9	3.3
Other	12	4.4

Attitudes

Tobacco attitudes increased from an average of 0.9 at Time 1 to 1.2 at Time 2 ($P < 0.01$). Marijuana attitudes increased from 1.9 at Time 1 to 2.3 at Time 2 ($P < 0.01$).

Intentions

Intention to use tobacco in the next 6 months increased from 0.4 at Time 1 to 0.8 at Time 2 ($P = 0.03$). Intention to use marijuana increased from 0.7 at Time 1 to 1.1 at Time 2 ($P < 0.01$). Table 2 summarizes attitude and intention data.

Table 2

Attitude & Intention Changes Reported by First-Year College Students

N=275	**Time 1: Prior to College**	**Time 2: After First Year of College**	***P*-value***
Tobacco Attitude	0.9	1.2	<0.01
Marijuana Attitude	1.9	2.3	<0.01
Tobacco Intention	0.4	0.8	0.03
Marijuana Intention	0.7	1.1	<0.01

**P*-value assessed using Wilcoxon signed-rank test for paired data

Behaviors

At Time 1, 15.0% of participants were current tobacco users and 15.7% were current marijuana users. The average age of first tobacco use was 16.8 years and the average age of first marijuana use was 16.5 years. Approximately one-third (32.0%) of college students had used tobacco before freshman year and 32.7% had used marijuana. After arriving at college, 12.2% of total participants initiated tobacco use ($P < 0.01$) while 13.5% initiated marijuana use ($P < 0.01$).

By the end of freshman year, 44.2% of total participants had used tobacco and 46.2% had used marijuana. At Time 2, 19.5% of participants were current tobacco users and 21.7% were current marijuana users. There was no significant difference in reported current use between Time 1 and Time 2 for either substance. Participants had used an average of 1.8 different tobacco consumption methods at Time 1 and an average of 2.1 at Time 2; participants had tried an average of 2.1 different marijuana consumption methods at Time 1 and an average of 3.8 at Time 2. Figures 1 and 2 summarize tobacco and marijuana consumption data.

FIGURE 1: Changes in Tobacco Methods of Consumption for First-Year College Students between Time 1 and Time 2

Legend – Figure 1	
	= # of participants at Time 1
	= # of participants at Time 2

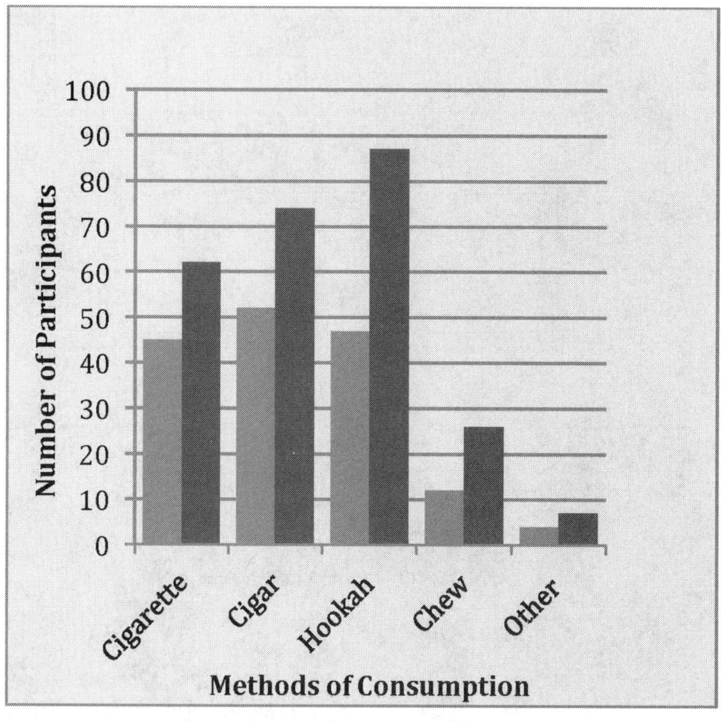

FIGURE 2: Changes in Marijuana Methods of Consumption for First-Year College Students between Time 1 and Time 2

Legend – Figure 2	
	= # of participants at Time 1
	= # of participants at Time 2

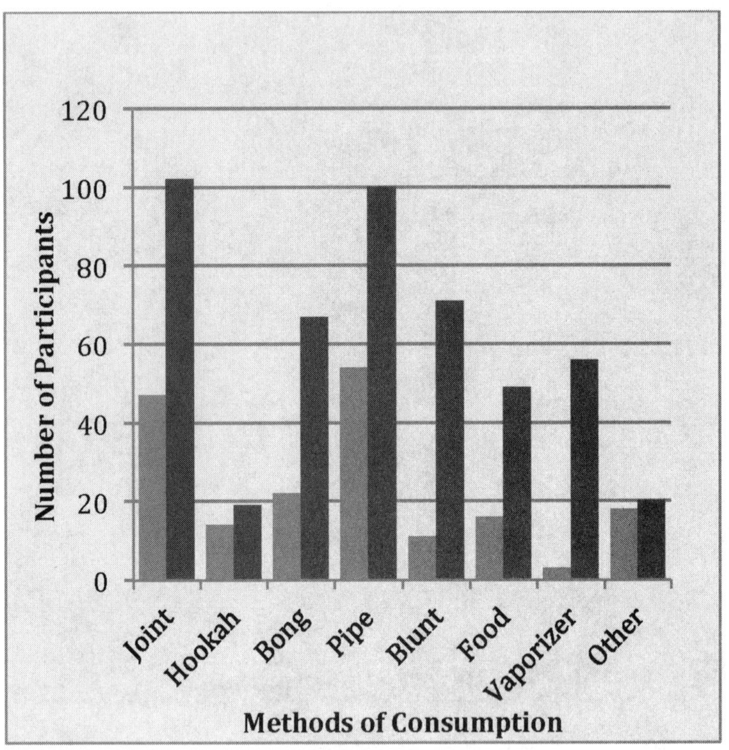

Multivariate Models

Model 1 assessed tobacco initiation. The 187 participants who reported no lifetime tobacco use at Time 1 were included in this model. Of this population, 38 participants initiated tobacco use by Time 2. Among tobacco initiators, initiation of tobacco use by Time 2 was positively associated with intention to use tobacco at Time 1 (OR = 2.1, 95% CI; 1.0-4.15, $P = 0.04$).

Model 2 assessed tobacco maintenance. The 88 participants who reported lifetime tobacco use at Time 1 were included in this model. Of these participants, 40 reported current tobacco use at Time 2. Among tobacco maintainers, positive intention was associated with current use at Time 2 (OR = 2.1, 95% CI; 1.2-3.5, $P = 0.008$).

Model 3 assessed marijuana initiation. The 185 participants who had never used marijuana at Time 1 were included in this model. At Time 2, 39 of these participants had initiated marijuana use. For marijuana initiators, initiation of marijuana by Time 2 was associated with both positive attitude at Time 1 (OR = 1.6, 95% CI; 1.1-2.4, $P = 0.02$) and intention (OR = 2.1, 95% CI; 1.2-3.5, $P = 0.007$).

Model 4 assessed marijuana maintenance. The 88 participants who reported lifetime marijuana use at Time 1 were included in this model. At Time 2, 44 of these participants reported current marijuana use. Among marijuana maintainers, neither attitude (OR = 0.9, 95% CI 0.5-1.6, $P = 0.8$) nor intention (OR = 1.2, 95% CI 0.7-2.04, $P = 0.4$) was associated with current use at Time 2. Figure 3 demonstrates these relationships.

FIGURE 3: Predictors of Tobacco and Marijuana Initiation and Maintenance during Students' First Year of College

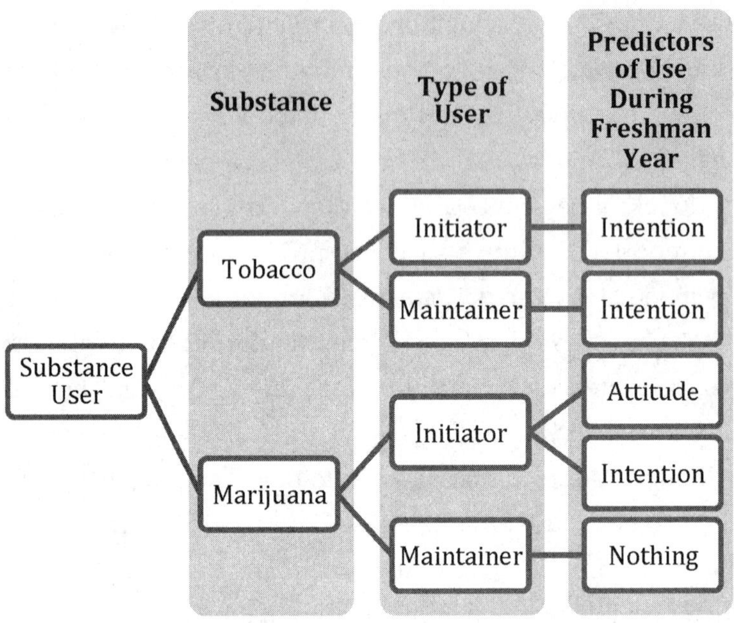

Discussion

Two important points can be gleaned from these results: (1) Attitudes, intentions, and behaviors toward tobacco and marijuana all change significantly toward favored use during students' first year of college, and (2) different mechanisms predict tobacco and marijuana initiation and continued use in this population, thereby suggesting a framework for targeted interventions.

Attitude, Intention, and Behavior Changes

Participants' attitudes toward, intentions to use, and actual use of both substances increased significantly during freshman year. Consistent with previous findings, external factors such as decreased adult supervision, increased availability and opportunity, or a sense of anonymity in the new community may all contribute to increased attitudes, intentions, and behaviors during this transition. [19] Further, social substance use, which is prevalent in the college setting,[10] may play a large role as students form new friendships and attempt to redefine their attitudes and intentions in the college environment.

Although attitudes toward and intentions to use both substances increased significantly during students' first year of college, it is interesting to note that both variables favored marijuana over tobacco. Attitudes toward tobacco at both Time 1 and Time 2 were less positive than attitudes toward marijuana at Time 1 alone. Further, intention to use marijuana was higher at both Time 1 and Time 2 than intention to use tobacco at the same times. Actual use of both substances reflects these attitudes and intentions, illustrating that marijuana was both initiated at a younger age and was more widely used among first-year college students in regard to overall and current use. Thus, results suggest that, compared to tobacco, there is a more widespread acceptance of marijuana use among college students. This trend parallels previous findings, which show a steadily rising rate of current marijuana use among 18 to 25-year-olds on a national scale.[30]

The prevalence of tobacco and marijuana use among the current study participants was higher than the national averages reported by the National College Health Association. About one-third of matriculating college students in the current study had already used one or both substances. By the end of their first year, nearly half of all students had tried one or both substances. These comparatively higher rates could be attributed to several factors, including an existing upward trend of substance use among this population as a whole, or to the population of students at the particular universities included in this study. Although cigarette smoking rates are historically low,[30] current findings illustrate that nicotine use in general is still common among first-year college students. Further, the current data corroborates prior research, showing that marijuana use among college students continues to increase.[3,30]

Methods of consumption became more varied across use of both substances. Hookah and cigars were the most popular methods of tobacco consumption. Because the hookah is designed for group use,[31] its rise in prevalence among this population may not be surprising. Further, this data shows that the hookah has surpassed cigarettes as the most popular method of tobacco consumption among college students. Consistent with other research findings, this suggests a trend toward social tobacco use during students' first year of college.[10]

Marijuana consumption methods also became more diversified. By the end of students' freshman year, joints were the most commonly used mode while bongs, blunts, marijuana in food, and vaporizers also increased in popularity. The average marijuana user had tried nearly four different methods by follow-up, suggesting that part of the appeal of marijuana use may be the myriad of ways in which it can be consumed. Similar to tobacco, methods of marijuana consumption that were conducive to social or multiple-person use became more popular. This may not be surprising, given that the main reasons college students cite for using marijuana relate to social facilitation.[32] Overall, freshman year represents a period of momentous change for students. Attitude, intention, and behavior changes toward tobacco and marijuana reflect just some of these vicissitudes.

Predictors of Use

Predictors of initiation or continuation of use differed by substance, suggesting that different prevention approaches may be beneficial for these two substances. Given the broad initiation of tobacco and marijuana use among first-year college students, there is compelling evidence that this population comprises an ideal target group for intervention.

The statistical models show that a student's intention to

use tobacco is the strongest predictor underlying both initiation and maintained use of the substance. This demonstrates that young adults generally have unfavorable attitudes toward tobacco, possibly because of exposure to televised antismoking advertisements or increased cost of tobacco products in the past decade.[33] Therefore, increased intentions and, consequently, increased propensity to use tobacco, may be attributable to factors such as social pressure rather than positive attitudes. Given the broad increase in social tobacco use during students' first year of college, "intention interventions" would have to be largely centered on targeting both the social conditions under which the behavior occurs and the negative social outcomes of the behavior.

Attitude and intention both predict marijuana initiation among first-year college students. Because there are fewer studies demonstrating possible long-term health effects of marijuana, it may be perceived as harmless or non-addictive. Further, marijuana's perceived conduciveness to social situations, along with its varying legal status, may make experimentation with the substance more appealing to young adults. Considering what is known about first-year students' perceptions of marijuana use on college campuses,[18] the belief that marijuana is "what everyone does" may also encourage students to try the substance. Through an understanding of the factors that predict initiation of marijuana during students' freshman year, interventions targeting both attitudes and intentions can be employed before life-long use is established.

This study is particularly relevant to current political debate surrounding both campus tobacco policies and marijuana legalization in the United States. The two universities in the current study have similar tobacco policies, which prohibit smoking in all buildings, vehicles, and facilities affiliated with the universities. This smoke-free policy also encompasses school dormitories and other residence halls, where the majority of college freshmen live. At the University of Wisconsin-Madison, students are allowed to smoke 25 feet from buildings and at the University of Washington-Seattle, there are designated outdoor locations for students to smoke. Within recent years, many college campuses in the United States have adopted total tobacco bans on all cigarettes and related products, which may impact tobacco use on those campuses. Similar policies for marijuana use may soon be implemented at the University of Washington-Seattle, where it is now legal for students over the age of 21 to use recreational marijuana. Undoubtedly, marijuana availability and consumption will continue to increase on college campuses following its legalization in different parts of the country. Therefore, the implications of this study may be especially pertinent to prevention and intervention efforts as tobacco bans are implemented and as marijuana gains legal status.

Limitations

This study presents several limitations. Given the similar demographics and lack of ethnic diversity of the two schools surveyed, the current data is not necessarily representative of all college campuses. We cannot guarantee perfect reliability or validity of the self-report scales or deny the possible presence of the social desirability bias. Further, while the statistical models showed strong associations between attitudes, intentions, and behaviors, causality cannot necessarily be drawn from these associations.

Further Studies

Additional studies are needed to determine attitudes, intentions, and behaviors among first-year college students across a larger sample of universities. While our study populations were representative of the ethnic diversity on each campus, there was an overall preponderance of Caucasians in the study. Future studies should investigate universities with a wider range of diversity. Examination of factors underlying changes in attitudes and intentions toward these substances is also warranted.

Acknowledgements

The authors would like to thank the Social Media and Adolescent Health Research Team for their help with data collection.

Funding sources

This study was supported by grant R01DA031580-03 which is supported by the Common Fund, managed by the OD/Office of Strategic Coordination (OSC).

Author Contributions

Conceived and designed the experiments: MAM, MWS.

Analysed the data: MAM, MWS. Wrote the first draft of the manuscript: MWS. Contributed to the writing of the manuscript: MWS, MAM. Agree with manuscript results and conclusions: MWS, MAM. Jointly developed the structure and arguments for the paper: MWS, MAM. Made critical revisions and approved final version: MWS, MAM.

Disclosures and Ethics

As a requirement of publication author(s) have provided to the publisher signed confirmation of compliance with legal and ethical obligations including but not limited to the following: authorship and contributorship, conflicts of interest, privacy and confidentiality and (where applicable) protection of human and animal research subjects. The authors have read and confirmed their agreement with the ICMJE authorship and conflict of interest criteria. The authors have also confirmed that this article is unique and not under consideration or published in any other publication, and that they have permission from rights holders to reproduce any copyrighted material. Any disclosures are made in this section. The external blind peer reviewers report no conflicts of interest.

References

1. Primack BA, Kim KH, Shensa A, Sidani JE, Barnett TE, Switzer GE. Tobacco, marijuana, and alcohol use in university students: a cluster analysis. *J Am Coll Health.* Jul 2012;60(5):374-386.

2. Results from the 2011 NSDUH: Summary of National Findings, SAMHSA, CBHSQ. 2012.

3. Meier MH, Caspi A, Ambler A, et al. Persistent cannabis users show neuropsychological decline from childhood to midlife. *Proc Natl Acad Sci U S A.* 2012.

4. Association ACH. American College Health Association National College Health Assessment II: Reference Group Executive Summary Fall 2011. In: Hanover MACHA, 2012, eds.

5. Pinchevsky GM, Arria AM, Caldeira KM, Garnier-Dykstra LM, Vincent KB, O'Grady KE. Marijuana exposure opportunity and initiation during college: parent and peer influences. *Prev Sci.* Feb 2012;13(1):43-54.

6. Sims TH, Abuse CoS. From the American Academy of Pediatrics: Technical report—Tobacco as a substance of abuse. *Pediatrics.* Nov 2009;124(5):e1045-1053.

7. Health CsOoSa. Smoking and Tobacco Use; Fact Sheet; Tobacco-Related Mortality. 2009; http://www.cdc.gov/tobacco/data_statistics/fact_sheets/health_effects/tobacco_related_mortality/.

8. Jacobsen LK, Krystal JH, Mencl WE, Westerveld M, Frost SJ, Pugh KR. Effects of smoking and smoking abstinence on cognition in adolescent tobacco smokers. 1 January 2005 2005;57(1):56–66.

9. Rigotti NA, Lee JE, Wechsler H. US college students' use of tobacco products: results of a national survey. *JAMA.* Aug 2000;284(6):699-705.

10. Moran S, Wechsler H, Rigotti NA. Social smoking among US college students. *Pediatrics.* Oct 2004;114(4):1028-1034.

11. Project MUSE The Role of Peer Relationships in Adjustment to College. 2012; http://muse.jhu.edu/journals/csd/summary/v049/49.6.swenson.html.

12. Johnston LD, O'Malley PM, Bachman JG, Schulenberg JE. Monitoring the Future national survey results on drug use, 1975-2011: Volume II, College students and adults ages 19-50.: Ann Arbor: Institute for Social Research, The University of Michigan; 2012.

13. Liu LY. 2005 Texas Survey of Substance Use Among College Students: Texas Department of State Health Services; 2007.

14. Hancox RJ, Poulton R, Ely M, et al. Effects of cannabis on lung function: a population-based cohort study. *Eur Respir J.* Jan 2010;35(1):42-47.

15. Zickler P. Marijuana Smoking Is Associated With a Spectrum Of Respiratory Disorders. *National Institute on Drug Abuse* 2006; http://www.drugabuse.gov/news-events/nida-notes/2006/10/marijuana-smoking-associated-spectrum-respiratory-disorders.

16. Gater P. Respiratory Effects of Marijuana. 2012; http://adai.uw.edu/marijuana/factsheets/respiratoryeffects.htm. Accessed July 19, 2012.

17. Gleason KA, Birnbaum SG, Shukla A, Ghose S. Susceptibility of the adolescent brain to cannabinoids: long-term hippocampal effects and relevance to schizophrenia. *Transl Psychiatry.* 2012;2:e199.

18. Gold GJ, Nguyen AT. Comparing entering freshmen's perceptions of campus marijuana and alcohol use to reported use. *J Drug Educ.* 2009;39(2):133-148.

19. Fromme K, Corbin WR, Kruse MI. Behavioral risks during the transition from high school to college. *Dev Psychol.* Sep 2008;44(5):1497-1504.

20. Wakefield MA, Loken B, Hornik RC. Use of mass media campaigns to change health behaviour. *Lancet.* Oct 9 2010;376(9748):1261-1271.

21. Campaign for Tobacco Free Kids. 2012; http://www.tobaccofreekids.org/what_we_do/state_local/taxes/.

22. Collins SE, Witkiewitz K, Larimer ME. The Theory of Planned Behavior as a Predictor of Growth in Risky College Drinking. Vol 72(2): J Stud Alcohol and Drugs; 2011:322-332.

23. Kam JA, Matsunaga M, Hecht ML, Ndiaye K. Extending the theory of planned behavior to predict alcohol, tobacco, and marijuana use among youth of Mexican heritage. *Prev Sci.* Mar 2009;10(1):41-53.

24. Ajzen I. The Theory of Planned Behavior. 1991; http://www.cas.hse.ru/data/816/479/1225/Oct%2019%20Cited%20%231%20Manage%20THE%20THEORY%20OF%20PLANNED%20BEHAVIOR.pdf.

25. D'Angelo J, Vander Heide J. The formation of physician credibility ratings in online communities: Negativity, Positivity and Non-normativity effectsIn press.

26. Hong S, Tandoc E, Jr., Kim EA, Kim B, Wise K. The real you? The role of visual cues and comment congruence in perceptions of social attractiveness from facebook profiles. *Cyberpsychol Behav Soc Netw.* Jul 2012;15(7):339-344.

27. Devos-Comby L, Lange JE. Standardized measures of alcohol-related problems: a review of their use among. *Psychol Addict Behav.* Sep 2008;22(3):349-361.

28. O'Callaghan F, Chang D, Callan V, Baglioni A. Models of alcohol use by young adults: an examination of various attitude-behavior theories. *Journal of Studies on Alcohol.* 1997;58(5):502-507.

29. Benevene P, Scopelliti M. Building a multi-dimensional scale on attitudes toward alcohol consumptions. *European Journal of Social Sciences.* 2012;34(1):58-69.

30. Results from the 2010 NSDUH: Summary of National Findings, SAMHSA, CBHSQ. 2012.

31. Akl EA, Gaddam S, Gunukula SK, Honeine R, Jaoude PA, Irani J. The effects of waterpipe tobacco smoking on health outcomes: a systematic review. 2010-06-01 2010.

32. Beck KH, Caldeira KM, Vincent KB, O'Grady KE, Wish ED, Arria AM. The social context of cannabis use: relationship to cannabis use disorders and depressive symptoms among college students. *Addict Behav.* Sep 2009;34(9):764-768.

33. Wakefield MA, Durkin S, Spittal MJ, et al. Impact of Tobacco Control Policies and Mass Media Campaigns on Monthly Adult Smoking Prevalence. Vol 98(8): American Journal of Public Health; 2008:1443-1450.

HAROLD KALANT CM, MD, PHD, FRSC
Professor Emeritus, University of Toronto,
Research Director Emeritus, Centre for Addiction and Mental Health

Marijuana: Medicine, Addictive Substance, or Both? A Common-Sense Approach to the Place of Cannabis in Medicine

The Canadian Journal of Addiction

THE EARLIER PLEBISCITE results in a number of American states that legalized use of "medical marijuana", and the more recent votes in favour of outright legalization of marijuana in Colorado and Washington, have naturally raised the question of whether the United States is moving inevitably towards full legalization, and whether Canada will be carried along by a tide of generational change. Speculation is further stimulated by the intention of Health Canada to change the ground rules of the Medical Marihuana Access Programme in a way that, superficially at least, looks like a move toward treating cannabis in the same way as other controlled medications. The proposal is to remove Health Canada from the business of controlling access to marijuana for medical use, and to allow physicians to write prescriptions that would be filled by licensed suppliers who would produce the drug in accordance with purity standards laid down by Health Canada.

A large majority of Canadian physicians appear to be very uneasy about this prospect, on the grounds that they lack sound scientific evidence about the therapeutic value of cannabis for different indications, about appropriate dosage, and about the balance of benefits and risks. Many also appear to be uneasy about the possibility of being exploited by non-medical users seeking to obtain the drug free of legal risks by pretending to have medical complaints requiring its use. This is an understandable fear, because experience in several American states that set up "medical marijuana" programs has shown that the most common complaint used to justify the issuance of marijuana access cards has been chronic back or neck pain in otherwise healthy young males (Nunberg et al., 2011; Reinarman et al. 2011). Nevertheless, there is indeed scientific evidence that cannabis, and some of the pure cannabinoids, do have potentially beneficial effects in certain disease processes. It is therefore important for physicians to have access to that information, and to know when they can justifiably use these agents therapeutically, and when they can or should not.

Crude cannabis had a long history of use as a medication in many parts of the world, but was perhaps best documented in India, where the Indian Hemp Drugs Commission examined its role in folk medicine in great detail (Kalant, 1972). From the mid-19th century onward, standardized extracts of cannabis found their way into the British and US Pharmacopoeias and were widely used in western medicine, often as components of multidrug mixtures prescribed as sedatives, anxiolytics, "tonics", cough syrups and other remedies. However, from the early 20th century on, such mixtures were soon displaced by new synthetic drugs of many kinds, with more selective actions, longer shelf life, and more accurately controllable dosage. Cannabis fell out of use in western medicine, and was eventually banned in most countries as part of the growing reliance on national and international drug control legislation that was originally designed to control traffic in opiates but was extended to include a broad range of other psychoactive agents.

The world-wide adoption of cannabis as part of the youth culture of the early 1970s was based on its mood and perception altering properties, which made it the "recreational drug" of choice for those who rejected conventional society and its use of alcohol. However, even though this was, and remains, the acknowledged principal role of cannabis, a significant percentage of those who became regular users claim that they use it at least in part for its beneficial effects on various physical or mental complaints (Ogborne et al., 2000). There was a notable similarity between the symptoms or diseases for which it had been used by mouth in Indian traditional medicine and those for which present-day marijuana smokers say they use it medically. Among both populations it was reported to relieve nausea and vomiting, pain, convulsive disorders, spasticity of both skeletal and smooth muscle, fever, depression, anxiety, sleeplessness and other symptoms, related to such diverse diseases as multiple sclerosis, glaucoma, epilepsy, HIV/AIDS and cancer (Russo, 2007). These claims were met with considerable skepticism by most medical practitioners, both because they were based largely on undocumented subjective claims by users, and because it was very difficult to conceive of a mechanism of action that could explain such widely differing therapeutic effects.

Such a mechanism has become scientifically validated only in recent years. After the discovery of the CB1 and CB2 cannabinoid receptors in the late 1980s, endogenous ligands that attached to these receptors were soon discovered and were named endocannabinoids, even though they are chemically different from the true cannabinoids found in the cannabis plant (phytocannabinoids). Additional receptors, such as GPR55, GPR 18 and TRPV1, were later found to bind not only endocannabinoids but also a variety of phytocannabinoids and synthetic analogs. The endocannabinoids, the enzymes that synthesize and degrade them, and the receptors to which they bind, are extremely widely distributed throughout the brain and most other tissues and organs of the body. They alter the movement of calcium and potassium ions across presynaptic membranes, and function as rapid but short-acting inhibitors of release of the conventional neurotransmitters from axon terminals, including those of glutamate, GABA, glycine, acetylcholine, noradrenaline, dopamine and serotonin neurons (Pertwee, 2009; Kalant, 2013). The extremely widespread distribution of the endocannabinoid system throughout the body, and its action on so many different neurotransmitters, explain how the cannabinoids are able to affect such a broad range of physical and mental functions, with both therapeutically useful and potentially harmful effects.

The harmful effects have in the past been studied and documented more thoroughly than the therapeutically useful ones (Kalant, 2004, 2013). Probably most physicians are aware of the impairment of learning, memory, alertness, reaction speed and judgment that are characteristic of acute intoxication with cannabis, and that result in impairment of school and work performance and of operation of aircraft and motor vehicles. Less well known is the inhibitory effect of chronic cannabis exposure on the maturation of neuronal pathways in the fetus and in childhood and early adolescence, with resulting mild but long-lasting impairment of so-called executive functions such as problem solving, comparative evaluation of alternative options, and working memory (Smith et al., 2010). Chronic smoking of cannabis, as distinct from the actions of cannabinoids *per se*, is also known to give rise to chronic inflammatory changes in the airways, with chronic cough and wheezing, and precancerous histological changes in the bronchial epithelium. It is important to note that most of the information about adverse effects has come from studies of heavy non-medical use of cannabis, not from therapeutic use of smaller amounts of cannabis or of pure cannabinoids. As with any drug therapy, therefore, it is necessary to think in terms of dose-response functions, and in the margin of safety that separates dose-response curves for the beneficial effects from those for harmful effects.

A number of the potentially useful effects have been well

studied and confirmed scientifically in both experimental animals and human volunteers and patients (Health Canada, 2013; Kalant, 2013). One of these is the moderately good analgesic action, principally against chronic musculoskeletal and neuropathic pain. Several clinical studies (e.g., Elikottil et al., 2009) have shown that combining smaller doses of cannabinoid and opioid can give good analgesic effect and fewer side effects than a larger dose of either drug alone. Cannabis, or pure Δ^9 –tetrahydrocannabinol (THC), can prevent or relieve nausea and vomiting induced by cancer chemotherapy or radiotherapy, and by drug treatment of HIV/AIDS. Stimulation of appetite and food intake in cachectic patients has also been demonstrated, but is of somewhat limited usefulness because cannabinoids increase mainly carbohydrate and fat intake, and not intake of protein that is needed for tissue regeneration. A moderate amount of scientific research on the role of the endocannabinoid system in the induction of REM and slow-wave sleep is also consistent with the long history of use of cannabis as a sedative and hypnotic. These therapeutic effects are usually, though not always, attainable with relatively small doses of cannabis or cannabinoids that do not result in serious adverse effects. In patients who have not had previous experience with cannabis, however, the margin of safety may be small. For example, in several studies of antiemetic and analgesic actions in cancer patients, a significant number of patients discontinued therapy because the desired effects were outweighed by unpleasant and disturbing effects such as mental clouding, anxiety and sense of unreality.

Other potential therapeutic effects of cannabis and certain pure cannabinoids have not proven to be clinically useful because the margin of safety has been clearly too small. This is true, for example, of the cannabis-induced lowering of intra-ocular pressure in glaucoma (Green, 1998), and the immunosuppressant action of cannabis and of Δ^9–THC that might otherwise have been useful in the treatment of autoimmune diseases or to prevent organ transplant rejection. An anticancer effect, consisting of inhibition of tumor cell growth *in vitro*, and of tumor vascularization, invasiveness and metastasis in a variety of animal models, is seen only at cannabinoid concentrations that are much higher than those attained systemically by even very heavy cannabis smokers.

Several other possible therapeutic applications still require more clinical study to determine whether they are practical, and if so, within what limits. One such possible use is in the treatment of spasticity in patients with multiple sclerosis. The prevailing opinion until recently was that cannabis relieves the subjective discomfort but does not alter objective measures of muscle spasticity (Zajicek and Apostu, 2011). However, a recent study (Corey-Bloom et al., 2012) found both subjective and objective improvement; clearly, further clinical trials are required. Inflammatory reactions, including osteoarthritis, chronic intestinal inflammatory disease, and the inflammatory component of posttraumatic or toxic brain damage (neuroprotective action), appear to be a promising target for cannabis/cannabinoid therapy, because the anti-inflammatory effect can also be produced by cannabinoids that do

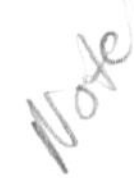

not act through the CB1 receptor and therefore do not produce the undesired cognitive and psychomotor disturbances (Guindon and Hohmann, 2008). Another possible application may be as an anticonvulsant agent in the treatment of some types of epilepsy. One early clinical study found that addition of cannabidiol (which is devoid of the unwanted psychoactive effects of THC) to the treatment regimen improved the seizure control in patients in whom conventional antiepileptic drugs had not given a satisfactory response (Cunha et al., 1980). However, other studies have given contradictory results, and more well-designed clinical trials are needed to establish whether cannabinoid therapy represents a useful addition, and if so, in which types of patient. There is a similar lack of sufficient evidence at present to support a number of other claimed uses of cannabis or cannabinoid therapy in such motor disorders as Parkinson's disease, Huntington's disease and Tourette's syndrome.

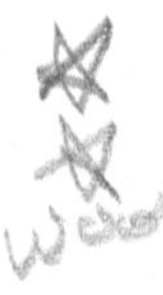

What positions can physicians reasonably adopt, therefore, when patients inquire about, or request, treatment with cannabis? A number of points can usefully be borne in mind, that can help to differentiate appropriate from inappropriate use. The first is that medical use and non-medical use have nothing whatever to do with each other. Heroin can be legally prescribed in Canada for relief of suffering in terminally ill cancer patients, yet no one suggests that heroin should therefore be available for non-medical use. There is no rational basis for thinking differently about cannabis. By prescribing it only for those who have a legitimate medical indication, and only in amounts appropriate for that indication, physicians should not fear that they are furthering the spread of illicit drug use. Health Canada (2013) provides detailed online information that can aid the physician in deciding what are the legitimate indications.

A second point is that cannabinoids are not the drugs of first choice for any of the medical complaints for which they may be used. For example, ondansetron and similar agents have more potent and longer-lasting antinauseant effect than THC, although smoking cannabis delivers a more rapid onset of action (Machado Rocha et al., 2008). However, some patients who fail to respond adequately to the preferred agents for a given indication may benefit from cannabis or cannabinoid therapy. Therefore, if a patient requests cannabis for what appears to be a legitimate medical reason, a preferred agent can be tried first and cannabis can be added or substituted only if the first agent does not give satisfactory results.

A third (and related) point is that the great majority of clinical studies have been done with THC or other pure cannabinoids given by mouth rather than with crude cannabis given by smoking. Though smoked cannabis has a more rapid onset of action, oral cannabinoids have a more even and longer sustained effect, and are therefore more convenient with respect to dosing schedule, as well as avoiding the risks of respiratory damage. They also produce lower peak concentrations which, in addition to their slower onset of action, contribute to their being less likely to give rise to dependence. In addition, pure THC (Marinol)* and nabilone (Cesamet) for oral use, and

Sativex (a standardized extract containing equal amounts of THC and cannabidiol) for sublingual spray, can be prescribed legally and dispensed by pharmacies in Canada, so that the physician need not fear being in contact with illegal substances. The claims frequently made by zealous users for the superior merits of one strain or another of cannabis for the treatment of different symptoms or diseases have no basis in scientific research, and can be disregarded by the physician.

A fourth point is that research on the endocannabinoid system is rapidly yielding new knowledge of its workings, and new agents for selectively modulating its activity in specific sites in the body (Baillie et al., 2013). It seems highly likely that in the near future a range of new drugs will become available that will provide desired cannabis-like effects in specific tissues and disease processes, without the unwanted side effects and problems that can be created by smoking crude cannabis. Therefore the physician can prescribe cannabis or cannabinoid therapy at present for those who can benefit from it, as an interim measure until superior agents become available. This may ease the professional concerns of those who are justifiably uneasy about the use of a crude product with much too broad a spectrum of effects. At the same time it will be incumbent on the physician to keep up to date with the evolving clinical literature, so that the interim measure can be replaced by the new agents as they arrive.

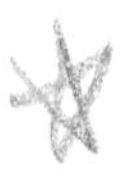

Finally, the physician has an obligation to screen carefully those patients who request cannabis therapy. For the developmental reasons described above, it should not be given to children or adolescents, nor to pregnant women. The experience in several American states cited above does indeed demonstrate the risk that many users of cannabis for non-medical purposes may request medical prescription of cannabis for highly dubious complaints. The physician who encounters such requests must probe carefully into the applicant's previous history of drug use (including alcohol and tobacco as well as illicit drugs), as part of the process of assessing which claims are truly medical, and which patients are most likely to use the medication as prescribed, and only for medical purposes. This is fundamentally no different from the care that physicians must take in prescribing opioids, benzodiazepines and other drugs that carry a risk of dependence, and need not deter the physician from using cannabis or cannabinoids when medical evidence suggests that they may be beneficial.

* Marinol Ò was recently withdrawn from the Canadian market by the manufacturer, for unstated reasons. It is not clear whether this is a temporary or a permanent withdrawal.

....

References

Baillie, G.L., Horswill, J.G., Anavi-Goffer, S., Reggio, P.H., Bolognini, D. et al. (2013) CB91) receptor allosteric modulators display both agonist and signaling pathway specificity. *Molecular Pharmacology*, 83; 322-338.

Corey-Bloom, J., Wolfson, T., Gamst, A., Jin, S., Marcotte, T.D. et al. (2012) Smoked cannabis for spasticity in multiple sclerosis: a randomized, placebo-controlled trial. *Canadian Medical Association Journal*, 184: 1143-1150.

Cunha, J.M., Carlini, E.A., Pereira, A.E., Ramos, O.L., Pimentel, C.L. et al. (1980) Chronic administration of cannabidiol to healthy volunteers and epileptic patients. *Pharmacology*, 21: 175-185.

Elikottil, J., Gupta, P. and Gupta, K. (2009) The analgesic potential of cannabinoids. *Journal of Opioid Management*, 5: 341-357.

Green, K. (1998) Marijuana smoking vs. cannabinoids for glaucoma therapy. *Archives of Ophthalmology*, 116: 1433-1437.

Guindon, J. and Hohmann, A.G. (2008) Cannabinoid CB2 receptors: A therapeutic target for the treatment of inflammatory and neuropathic pain. *British Journal of Pharmacology*, 153: 319-334.

Health Canada (2013) Author: H. Abramovici. Cannabis (marihuana, marijuana) and the Cannabinoids. February, 2013 (pdf version) at www.hc-sc.gc.ca, Drugs & Health Products> Information for Health Care Professionals.

Kalant, H. (2004) Adverse effects of cannabis on health: an update of the literature since 1996. *Progress in Neuro-Psychopharmacology and Biological Psychiatry*, 28: 849-863.

Kalant, H. (2013) Effects of cannabis and cannabinoids in the human nervous system. In: *The Effects of Drug Abuse on the Human Nervous System*; B. Madras and M.J. Kuhar (Eds.), 2013 (in press), Elsevier, Amsterdam.

Kalant, O.J. (1972) Report of the Indian Hemp Drugs Commission, 1893-94: A critical review. *International Journal of the Addictions*, 7: 77-96.

Machado Rocha, F.C., Stefano, S.C., De Cassia Haiek, R., Rosa Oliveira, L.M.Q. and Da Silveira, D.X. (2008) Therapeutic use of Cannabis sativa on chemotherapy-induced nausea and vomiting among cancer patients. Systematic review and meta-analysis. *European Journal of Cancer care*, 17: 431-443.

Nunberg, H., Kilmer, B., Pacula, R.L. and Burgdorf, J.R. (2011) An analysis of applicants presenting to a medical marijuana specialty practice in California. *Journal of Drug Policy Analysis*, 4(1): 1-16. DOI: 10.2202/1941-2851.1017.

Ogborne, A.C., Smart, R.G. and Adlaf, E.M. (2000) Self-reported medical use of marijuana: A survey of the general population, *Canadian Medical Association Journal*, 162: 1685-1686.

Pertwee, R.G. (2009) Emerging strategies for exploiting cannabinoid receptor agonists as medicines. *British Journal of Pharmacology*, 156: 397-411.

Reinarman, C., Nunberg, H., Lanthier, F. and Heddleston, T, (2011) Who are medical marijuana patients? Population characteristics from nine California assessment clinics. *Journal of Psychoactive Drugs*, 43: 128-135.

Russo, E.B. (2007) History of cannabis and its preparations in saga, science and sobriquet. *Chemistry and Biodiversity*, 4: 1614-1648.

Smith, A.M., Longo, C.A., Fried, P.A., Hogan, M.J. and Cameron, I. (2010) Effects of marijuana on visuospatial working memory: an fMRI study in young adults. Psychopharmacology, 210: 429-438.

Zajicek, J.P. and Apostu, V.I. (2011) Role of cannabinoids in multiple sclerosis. *CNS Drugs*, 25: 187-201.

Reprinted with permission. *The Canadian Journal of Addiction*. September 2013.

Dr. Harold Kalant completed training for his MD degree in 1944, while serving in the RCAMC, and later had three years of postgraduate training in Internal Medicine at hospitals in Toronto, Saskatoon, and Santiago (Chile). In 1955 he obtained his PhD in Pathological Chemistry from the University of Toronto, followed by a postdoctoral fellowship in Biochemistry at the University of Cambridge, U.K. His previous positions were as Biochemistry Section Head, Defence Research Medical Laboratories, and then joint appointment as Associate Professor and later full Professor of Pharmacology, University of Toronto, and Associate Research Director. He was also Research Director, Biobehavioral Studies, at the Addiction Research Foundation of Ontario. Since 1989 he has been Professor Emeritus at the University of Toronto, and Research Director Emeritus at the Centre for Addiction and Mental Health. He has been an invited expert witness on alcohol and drug problems before committees of the governments of Canada and Ontario, and served as Chair or member of scientific advisory committees to CCSA, WHO, NIAAA, NIDA, and the Addiction Research Foundation of California. He has chaired two Expert Advisory Committees to Health Canada on medical uses of cannabis, and a World Health Organization working group on effects of cannabis on health. He has received many international honours, most recently, Member of the Order of Canada. His main areas of research and publication have been biological mechanisms of tolerance and dependence on alcohol, anxiolytics, opioids, and cannabis; their adverse effects on health; medical uses of cannabis and cannabinoids; and the role of science in drug policy. He and his late wife, Dr. Oriana Josseau Kalant, authored the book *Drugs, Society and Personal Choice* as a contribution to public discussion preceding the LeDain Commission report. Dr.Kalant sits on the advisory council of SAM Canada.

ROBERT B.
Former Assistant Secretary of State, US State Department's Bureau of International Narcotics and Law Enforcement Affairs

Finding Solutions

Unlikely Options: The Need to Avoid Recklessness

While it may seem obvious to some, the notion of standing by while narcotic traffickers and terrorists become more closely aligned is more than just reckless—it is certain to accelerate acts of terrorism and narcotics distribution. Neither outcome is one that Americans should want for themselves, their families, their communities, their nation, or the global community. Action is therefore the only real choice. But *what* action?

Before we get there, consider the other easy way out, one that seems to gain more glib adherents every day: Why not simply legalize narcotics—remove all legal restrictions on production and sale, as well as penalties—and, in the words of the eager few, "take the profit out of drug trafficking"?

Common Sense Against Legalizing Narcotics

Now *there* would be a neat trick—vanquishing an entire class of crime by making them legal! If it would work for narcotics, then why not for robbery, burglary, rape, and homicide? More seriously, do we really want the government to be in the business of "trafficking" or administering dangerous and destructive drugs? For whom would such drugs be legal—just adults? Who would pay for the explosive increase in social costs associated with predictable increases in use?

Who would cover the sudden spike in overdoses, emergency-room incidents, underweight births, infectious diseases, drug treatment programs, auto and workplace accidents, reduced labor productivity, lower educational achievement, crimes committed under the influence of drug use and addiction, elevated family dysfunction, increased domestic and child abuse—and human heartbreak?

Even more simply: Why wouldn't the legal drug market be subject to the same forces as every other legal market? How would legalization end the inevitable demand for purer and cheaper drugs—and more of them—than the government was willing to provide? Or the inevitable black market for narcotics below the government's "go-ahead-and-use" or "go-ahead-and-get-addicted" age? Or the obvious market for drugs so dangerous that even the government would not sanction their use? Or control over the various markets dominated by those outside the United States? In short, who would control the multilevel, still illegal, markets? The answer is the same people who control them today—drug traffickers and terrorist organizations—but with the difference that the American (and perhaps the European) markets would be *larger*. As more Americans tried these addictive substances, more would become addicted, a course extremely difficult to reverse once availability drives up use, elevating the aggregate number of people annually becoming addicted.

The end result would be a very sick nation, young and old, but one with enough wealth to keep buying until the combination of internal societal breakdown (economic and moral) and external threats, including terrorists flush with more drug money, brought the whole sad chapter to an end.

No—applying the principles of common sense, legalizing addictive drugs would not be prudent government. It would be reckless or, worse, an open invitation to national demise. We need not wander that dark alley, since formal economics suggests answers elsewhere.

Formal Economics Against Legalizing Narcotics

Okay, buckle up. Here we go. In formal economic terms, the central problem with drug legalization can be expressed as follows:

Every consumer of an addictive substance begins with a *first use* of that substance. That decision is informed by the cost of use, including price, risk of addiction and other perceived adverse health effects, and perceived benefits of use. As the consumer migrates from treating an addictive substance (for example, cocaine, heroin, marijuana) as a "luxury" to treating the same substance as a "necessity," substantial research indicates that the "price elasticity of demand" (PED) for the drug shrinks—that is, price has less of an effect on the decision to use.

Unlike the first-time user of drugs, who is assumed to have weighed the addictive substance's putative effects against costs and risks, often based on information (accurate and inaccurate) collected from peers, media, parents, and the community at large, an addicted person's decision-making is circumscribed by his or her addiction. The addicted person's role as a purchaser or consumer is quickly *defined by* his or her addiction.

The laws of supply and demand, requiring rational economic or consumer behavior, do not work when applied to the addicted consumer, to whom price becomes less important. Consistent with the clinically proven elements of addiction, including dependence and tolerance, the market as applied to this consumer is no longer characterized by free and rational choice. The PED has fallen to a low point; large changes in price do not affect the addicted person's demand for the addictive substance or commodity.

Now, where does that leave the legalization option? We can expect a few simple outcomes from policy choices that lead this way, whether they comprehend full legalization or merely a reduction in penalties. Policies that lower the price of addictive substances tend to increase first-time use, or initiation rates, for these substances. Increased use or initiation rates tend to increase addiction rates, based on the responsiveness of first-time and casual users to lower prices. All this assumes an unchanged quantity, but legalizing such substances (or lowering penalties for use and addiction) would increase availability, accelerating both use and addiction.

We can also say that, while raising prices of an addictive substance appears to lower the rate of first-time use or initiation for most addictive substances, higher prices do not appear to have any substantial impact on consumption by an already addictive population. Substitution of one addictive substance for another (similarly addictive) substance by an addicted population appears more likely at higher prices or in the event of lower availability. At the same time, "substitution" might include accessible, affordable treatment to end the addiction, when such an option is available; this is less likely to occur where significant effort is required by an addicted person to obtain treatment necessary to end the addiction.

In the end, rational or "free" choice by the addicted population appears to be significantly impaired by a combination of the cognitive deficit produced by using addictive substances (i.e., cognitive changes in brain function developing as a result of use of the addictive substance) and what is generally described as compulsion, a combination of dependence and growing tolerance to the addictive substance. Finally, there is this: Most discussants of legalization or government distribution of addictive substances do not take into account either (1) the predictable long-term growth in the population of addicted persons, or (2) the long-term addiction costs associated with the varying degrees of this policy choice.

In everyday terms, which economists seldom use, these ideas can be illustrated simply. The first rule is: Narcotics invariably slide down the so-called "price-elasticity scale"—starting as a luxury and ending up a necessity. This rule may be illustrated by an analogy.

Marijuana, cocaine, and heroin are highly addictive substances, whereas baseball games, carnival rides, and cotton candy are not. If prices rise on baseball tickets, carnival rides, or cotton candy—especially if the price rise is substantial—then buyers do not buy. Similarly, if prices are high for drugs, *first –time* purchasers act in the same way as nonaddicted buyers would act for any nonaddictive commodity, such as baseball, carnival tickets, or cotton candy: They do not buy.

On the other hand, regardless of increases in price, *addicted* persons exhibit far less freedom—if any—not to buy. Physiological and psychological dependencies dictate that higher prices will not deter buying or consuming. Data from both addictive science and criminal justice support this conclusion. Accordingly, drug addicted persons do not choose *not* to buy drugs as prices rise, since that is typically no longer viewed as an option.

So while lower prices might spur buying of drugs by nonaddicted persons and higher prices appear to reduce first-time buying among nonaddicts, there is strong evidence that higher prices to do not reduce buying by increasingly addicted persons. The implications of this argument are simply put: If narcotics of any kind were legalized, based on the addictive nature of these substances, several economic effects could be accurately predicted from low PEDs associated with these substances among addicted persons.

First, lower prices would drive a wider number of initial users to consume these substances. Estimates by economists range upward from 8 percent of the population who, for purely economic reasons, would begin to use at the lower prices created by legalization.

Even those economic thinkers who advocate legalization of addictive substances seem to concede that prices would fall and availability would rise. *The Economist*, for example, conceded in July 2001 that legalizing narcotics "would increase the number of people who took them, whatever restrictions were applied," on top of raising "difficult questions about who should distribute them and how." Still, many advocates seem unmoved by the argument that initiation rates will increase. There seems little concern that the PED for any *one* of countless addictive narcotics would rapidly slide from high to low as addiction spread. Even *The Economist*, which has elsewhere advocated such an approach, accepts this fact:

The number of drug users would rise for three reasons. First, the price of legalized drugs would almost certainly be lower—probably much lower—than the present price of illegal ones… Second, access to legalized drugs would be easier… And third, the social stigma against the use of drugs—which the law today helps to reinforce—would diminish. Many more people might try drugs if they did not fear imprisonment or scandal.[1]

Initially, this would amount to a new wave of freely made decisions, based on the information available from a variety of sources. The initial decision to use by these nonusers would weigh perceived costs and benefits, and produce, in some percentage of the population, a decision to begin use of the narcotic. Even conservative estimates of the percentage of first-time purchasers likely to become addicted, shows an enormous—some would say ominous—spike. The number of users and impact of legalization on addiction rates, objectively measurable social costs, and even such banal factors as state budgets, would be enormous. For these reasons, the narcotics legalization option is simply not an option—even in purely economic terms, it is a nonstarter.

Individually, we may not sit at the United Nations, work at the State Department, speak a foreign language, serve in Congress or a state legislature, or be able to tell the President of the United States (or any other country) just how much we think this issue matters; but we *can* talk about it with peers, parents, teachers, community leaders, and maybe even our congressional representatives. We can say, "Hey, this issue matters to us, as Americans." In the end, we can tackle some problems as individuals, more as families and communities, and still a larger number as a nation. This is one issue that will call out the best from all civilized members of the international community, if we are to sever the relationship between violent drug traffickers and ruthless terrorist organizations.

Finally, better drug treatment options for those Americans who have been caught in the spiderweb of addiction, there to languish without help, are needed. Though there is insufficient room here to discuss this vital topic in the detail it deserves, consider simply Ralph Waldo Emerson's observation that "every man is an empire." No one should be left behind in our national effort to stop the destructive forces of drug addiction and terrorism. Those caught in the web of addiction must be freed, even as we collectively fight to free and protect our nation. In practical terms, this means that we must see the pain of addiction as it is. Addiction affects individuals, families, communities, and the nation. We must be proactive in reaching out to those who suffer, consciously bringing along members of society who need our help, if we are to make the society itself healthier, safer, and more predictably secure.

No act by our government or by a terrorist can ever relieve us of the individual responsibility to do the right thing. Whether that requirement is in the context of defending the nation or defending an ideal in casual conversation, whether that reality triggers the need to write your congressional representative, start a community coalition, assist a friend, or steer clear of some action, the point remains the same. Whether in times of war or peace, at home, school, work, or recreation, the obligation of citizens to exercise individual responsibility for their own actions and to assist others in the society is paramount. In a time of national stress, the obligation is still higher.

Central to the link between narcotics and terrorism is one last, nagging fact: As a nation, we must be willing to project ourselves around the globe diplomatically and militarily, but also to pry ourselves from the sources of terrorist funding we have grown accustomed to overlooking. Only by seeing this link, understanding its significance, and taking a stand against it can we hope to free ourselves from two of the greatest threats this nation has ever faced: narcotics and terrorism. You now know the incontrovertible links, the logic behind the links, and the urgency of the national need to move forward with open eyes, acting on the best information available, to make wise decisions on a treacherous sea.

Together, narcotics traffickers and terrorists present a formidable adversary. Nevertheless, Americans can defeat them both and restore security, health, and safety to our homes, communities, and the nation. Terrorists, funded by drug money, represent a predator much like a shark. The lethality of the jaws depends directly on the support of the dorsal fin. Absent the dorsal fin, the shark flounders. We can end the parallel connection between terrorism and drugs by acknowledging the connection's existence, refusing to accept it, and acting to separate the jaws from the fin. In such a world, we all swim more safely in.

References

1 "Set It Free," *The Economist* (July28, 2001) pp. 15-16.

Robert B. Charles rejoined The Charles Group, LLC as President in April, 2005 after serving from 2003 to 2005 as Assistant Secretary of State, for International Narcotics and Law Enforcement Affairs (INL).

He founded The Charles Group, LLC in 1999 upon leaving service as Staff Director and Chief Counsel for the National Security, International Affairs, and Criminal Justice Subcommittee (GRO) in the House of Representatives from 1995–1999. Charles also served Subcommittee Chairman J. Dennis Hastert, onetime Speaker of the House, as chief staffer to The Speaker's Task Force on a Drug Free America from 1997-1999 and as top staffer to the Bi-Partisan Drug Policy Group from 1995-1999.

A former litigator in New York and Washington, Charles worked at Weil Gotshal & Manges and Kramer Levin between 1988 and 1995, clerked on the U.S. Court of Appeals for the Ninth Circuit, and taught both Government Oversight and Cyberlaw at Harvard University Extension School from 1998-2001. In 2000, he was awarded Harvard's prestigious Petra T. Shattuck Award for Excellence in Teaching by the University.

He authored *Narcotics and Terrorism*, a 2004 volume explaining national security and homeland security implications inherent in the worldwide illicit drug trade.

Charles received his J.D. from Columbia Law School in New York, M.A. in Politics, Philosophy and Economics from Oxford University in England, and A.B. from Dartmouth College in New Hampshire.

KALE PAULS RCMP

DR. IRWIN M. COHEN
University of the Fraser Valley

DR. DARRYL PLECAS
Professor Emeritus, School of Criminology and Criminal Justice,
Univsersity of the Fraser Valley

TARA HAARHOFF RCMP

The Nature and Extent of Marijuana Posession in British Columbia

Introduction

The illegal status of marihuana has been the subject of debate for decades. Quantitative accounts of the police response to marihuana possession offences using data from Statistics Canada are frequently quoted in the media, by advocate groups, political parties, policy makers, police, and by academics to support their positions. However, there is very little discussion or analyses into the challenges associated with the way Statistics Canada collects and reports this data. The purpose of this article is to examine marihuana possession offences in British Columbia from the number of recorded police seizures of marihuana to the number of individuals who received a criminal conviction for the offence in order to argue that the information reported in the media and used by many researchers vastly overestimates the number of people charge, convicted, and incarcerated for marihuana possession in British Columbia from 2009 to 2011.

The Vancouver Sun (2012) stated that marihuana possession charges in British Columbia were up 88% over the last decade; a policy paper by the federal Liberal Party of Canada (2013) stated in relation to marihuana "in some jurisdictions possession is prosecuted vigorously" and "across Canada 28,183 people were charged with possession of marijuana [in 2011]"; a recent study by Simon Fraser University Professor Neil Boyd (2013) stated that, in 2011, there were 3,774 charges for marihuana possession in British Columbia of which about 1,200 resulted in a conviction. In all cases, the data from these claims derived from Statistics Canada and are fundamentally incorrect or misleading.

The use of information from Statistics Canada has influenced those who create Canadian drug laws. In 1997, the two federal legislative branches created the Special Committee on Illegal Drugs designed to review all Canadian drug legislation. After a number of delays, the committee concluded in September 2002 with a final report titled, *Cannabis: Our Position for a Canadian Public Policy*. Using Statistics Canada data, they highlighted that, in 1999, there were approximately 50,000 drug related charges in Canada, of which 21,381 (43 per cent) were for the possession of cannabis. The committee discussed the implications this had for Canadians in relation to the principles of fairness and justice. Furthermore, the Office of the Auditor General of Canada (2001) used the same statistic in their report. Although the Auditor General recognized that drug data in general was sparse, often outdated, not available, or located in a myriad of different sites, it still made an estimate of the impact that the reported drug charges had on the court system. The caution that the Auditor General recognized in the recording for drug offence data appears to have not been responded to, and academics, drug policy advocates, politicians, police, and the media have continued to use the data from Statistics Canada to draw conclusions about the nature and extent of marihuana possession in British Columbia, and more broadly in Canada.

Statistics Canada obtain their data through mandatory reporting by police agencies across Canada. In British Columbia, all police agencies use a computerized records system called Police Records Information Management Environment (PRIME). PRIME captures the information required by the Canadian Centre for Justice Statistics (CCJS) through the Uniform Crime Reporting (UCR) surveys. In turn, the CCJS provides the data to Statistics Canada for their analysis and publishing.

In order to fully understand how marihuana possession offence statistics are gathered and tallied, a basic understanding of the Uniform Crime Reporting Survey is required. According to Statistics Canada (2012), the UCR was designed to measure the incidence of crime in Canadian society and its characteristics. The primary data used is in relation to incidents that the police have categorized as 'founded' meaning that the police have reason to believe that the offence actually took place. The UCR survey only captures the most serious offence of each eligible founded file on PRIME. Importantly, the UCR survey is incident based, not violation based. Given this, the status of the file is reflective of the entire incident and not each offence that may make up the incident. Furthermore, if one violation is cleared by charge or otherwise, the UCR survey records the entire incident as cleared. In the example of an assault offence and a marihuana offence being part of the same incident, the entire file is cleared if any one of these offences is cleared. However, the UCR survey rules state that traffic[1] and non-traffic incidents are to be scored as separate incidents. In the case of an impaired driver who was also in possession of marihuana, two police files should be generated; one to record the criminal traffic offence and one to record the drug offence (non-traffic offence). Moreover, if the police issued a violation ticket for a liquor act offence and, in the course of dealing with the subject, marihuana was located, but dealt with by way of a verbal warning, this would be recorded as a single incident with a cleared by charge status. In this case, the primary UCR code reported to CCJS would misrepresent the marihuana possession as cleared by charge.

Through the reporting to CCJS by each police agency, Statistics Canada provides annual reports on various offences, including drug offences. For 2011, the raw numbers from Statistics Canada state that police reported more than 113,164 drug offences in Canada. Of these, 61,406 (54 per cent) were for possession of marihuana. However, in this case, Statistics Canada used raw data from police where a seizure of marihuana was made, but this is not reflective of whether the

1 Within the meaning of the UCR survey, traffic and non-traffic offences refer to driving offences and non-driving offences and not drug trafficking.

police associated the marihuana to a person. Additionally, the number does not reveal anything about the action taken by police against any person that possessed marihuana.

According to Statistics Canada, in 2011, there were 3,774 people charged with possession of marihuana in British Columbia (see Table 1). Furthermore, a British Columbia Ministry of Justice (2012: 6) report emphasized, "the overall drug crime rate is driven by possession offences, specifically cannabis possession, which constitutes the majority of all drug offences". The report utilized Statistics Canada data to show that, in 2011, police recorded 16,578 founded marihuana possession offences, which included cleared and not cleared incidents, that 79% of these founded cases were cleared, but only 23% resulted in a person being charged with possession of marihuana. Although the overall number of incidents consistently increased from 2009 to 2011, the proportion of persons charged with marihuana possession over those three years remained constant.

TABLE 1: *Total Number of Marihuana Possession Offences and Number of Persons Charged in BC*

Type of Call	2009	2010	2011
Total Number of Founded Marihuana Possession Incidents in BC	13,284	15,721	16,578
Number of Incidents Cleared in BC	10,238	12,474	13,095
Number of Persons Charged with Marihuana Possession in BC	3,246	3,626	3,774

It is important to comprehend the definitions of the terms cleared and charged as used by Statistics Canada to understand the meaning of the data. An incident is cleared when the police have identified at least one offender in relation to an offence and have sufficient evidence to solve the offence (Mahony and Turner, 2010). An incident is cleared by charge when the police have sworn a charge or recommended a charge to Crown Counsel in relation to any offence that comprised the incident. In Canada, a formal accusation is made when an Information has been sworn to the court accusing a person of a specific offence, which initiates further proceedings by the court. In British Columbia, an Information is sworn, in most cases, on the approval of Crown Counsel after they have received the facts of the case from police and agree to proceed with the matter in court. Accordingly, in cases that are cleared by charge, it may be expected that not all incidents will proceed to court as Crown may quash the police laid charge or not approve a recommended charge.

Statistics Canada has a more liberal definition of charged stating that an offence is cleared by charge when either a charge has been laid (Information sworn) or a charge is recommended by police against at least one person on the police file. Another category of a founded police reported incident is cleared otherwise. CCJS states that for a file to be coded as cleared otherwise, which is sometimes referred to as cleared by other means, there must be sufficient evidence to lay a charge, but, for some reason, the police decide not to lay the charge. Common reasons for not charging can be: issuing a warning from police or using 'departmental discretion'; a complainant declines to press charges, which is not common to drug investigations as the police are typically the witness to the offence; the subject is already in prison and the current charge will not achieve any sentencing or criminal justice goals; or the case is referred to a diversion program. Hollins (2007) and McCormick et al. (2010) observed that the use of the cleared otherwise designation is inconsistent between jurisdictions making it extremely problematic to compare different jurisdictions' clearance rates.

To date, all the available literature regarding the nature of marihuana possession has relied on the charged data from Statistics Canada. As demonstrated in Table 1, in British Columbia, this suggests that 3,774 people in 2011 were charged with simple marihuana possession. However, no one has challenged the meaning of this figure despite its implication that, on average, 10 people per day in British Columbia are charged with possession of marihuana. Moreover, a review of court registry lists in British Columbia reveals a near absence of simple marihuana possession cases. This raises several important questions about the methods used to document the disposition of marihuana offences. To investigate this issue, all the police files in British Columbia with a marihuana possession UCR code for the years 2009 to 2011 were analyzed, including the court outcome and criminal record of those convicted, to provide an in-depth assessment of the nature and extent of marihuana possession in British Columbia.

Research Methodology

The methodology for determining the frequency of specific offences was to use the UCR code reported to CCJS by individual police agencies. As discussed in the previously mentioned studies and publications analyzing marihuana possession offences, researchers typically rely exclusively on the charged categorization for their analysis and do not investigate further into the nature of the charges (Boyd, 2013; Special Committee on Illegal Drugs, 2002). As a result, in this study, not only were the categorizations used by CCJS considered, but the primary files were consulted to provide more context to the data and allow for an analysis of the data without the definitional and criteria constraints imposed by CCJS reporting.

This study used anonymized data for the years 2009 to 2011 obtained from the RCMP through the University of the Fraser Valley RCMP Research Chair. The data included police incidents for each year that had as one of the four possible UCR offence codes; (1) Possession Cannabis Over 30 grams (4140-1), Possession—Cannabis 30 grams & Under (4140-2), Possession—Cannabis Resin Over 1 gram (4140-3), and Possession-Cannabis Resin 1 Gram & Under (4140-4). The data was collected from all municipal police agencies and RCMP detachments in BC from the PRIME database. To begin, the total number of marihuana possession files, including incidents where no marihuana was ever seized, was assessed. This included assistance files and files where a complaint was made regarding the possession of marihuana, but the police were either unable to verify the presences of it or they were able to verify through investigation that no marihuana was possessed. These assistance, unfounded, and unsubstantiated files are not relevant to actual police seizures of marihuana and were eliminated from the database leaving only founded incidents. In all founded cases, it was determined that marihuana was possessed, but this does not necessarily mean that it was associated to a person. Incidents where the marihuana was not associated to a person can include marihuana located in found property or marihuana turned over to the police by other agencies, such as schools, where no suspect name is known or provided. These cases are scored as founded—not cleared. Again, the founded—not cleared files do not offer any details about offenders and the file is primarily made as a mechanism to report and process the marihuana for destruction.

The two CCJS statuses used for marihuana possessed by a known person in which the police believe there is an offence contrary to the Canadian Controlled Drugs and Substances Act (CDSA) are founded—cleared otherwise and founded—cleared by charge. In the case of incidents scored as founded—cleared otherwise, this typically refers to the police taking no action against the person found in possession or the police issuing a verbal warning. In the case of a verbal warning, the incident is coded as founded—cleared otherwise: departmental discretion, as the officer uses their discretion to not proceed with an enforcement action. In the case of founded—cleared by charge incidents, it is implied that the police have proceeded against a person for illegal possession of marihuana or some other offence associated to the incident.

As it related to marihuana possession, all previous research stops the data dissection once it reaches the number of cases that were founded – cleared by charge. However, when the founded – cleared by charge files are examined, practitioners and researchers need to be cognizant of the broad interpretation of this status. As this study searched all PRIME files for a marihuana possession UCR code present in one of the four available UCR codes, the cleared by charge status may reflect the outcome of another offence. To assist in deciphering if the cleared by charge status is associated to the marihuana offence, an examination of the number of CDSA charges formally laid was conducted. The PRIME tracking of CDSA charges laid does not distinguish by the type of drug charge; therefore, the results may be referring to marihuana, cocaine, heroin, or some other drug. To assist in distinguishing the marihuana charges from the other drug charges, a search of PRIME files with only a marihuana possession charge as the UCR code was completed. This eliminated the possibility that any other criminal offence or drug offence could be the reason for the cleared by charge CCJS code. UCR survey rules state that a traffic offence and a non-traffic offence have to be scored as separate occurrences even though they are part of the same incident. Therefore, if scored properly by the police, some marihuana possession only files may be part of an impaired driving or other traffic offence. This would be very difficult to determine without reading each file narrative.

The total number of CDSA files that included marihuana possession as one of its four UCR codes was further broken down into the type of disposition of the CDSA charge. To organize the data, a total of 20 distinct dispositions or status categories were developed. This list was collapsed to combine similar dispositions into a common category. The final data extract involved reviewing all convictions for the CDSA offences and extracting the incidents that resulted in a prison sentence. The CPIC criminal records of persons sentenced to a period of incarceration for marihuana possession were examined from a random sample of 155 incidents. The records were coded separating variables for type of previous conviction, the length of an offender's criminal history, the length of any previous prison sentences, whether the offender met the designation of a prolific offender, and general demographic information. It should be noted that this methodology presents several limitations, including the fact that the researchers could not independently verify the validity or accuracy of the data. As is common practice, those who use CCJS data must rely on the clearance categories assigned without any external validation. Specifically on this point, McCormick et al. (2010) suggested that clearance rate statistics should be considered and used with caution, as there is widely inconsistent use of these categories by police.

Research Results

Between 2009 and 2011, there was an increase in the total number of files that had a marihuana possession UCR code in any of the four fields designated for an offence code. Specifically, the count increased from 18,961 in 2009 to 21,423 in 2010, to 22,561 in 2011. The total file count for each year included assistance files, unsubstantiated, and unfounded files, in addition to the founded files directly relevant to this study (see Table 2). An assistance file is typically a request from another detachment to assist in some way on an investigation, such as serving a summons or interviewing a witness. An unsubstantiated file includes reports made to police that, when investigated, it was determined that there was insufficient information to conclude that the offence occurred. An unfounded file includes reports made to police where an investigation has concluded that the offence did not occur.

TABLE 2: *Categorization of CCJS Code on PRIME for Files with Marihuana Possession*

CCJS Code	2009	2010	2011
Assistance, Unsubstantiated, and Unfounded	4,366	4,148	4,355
Founded – Not Cleared	3,122	3,432	3,370
Founded – Cleared Otherwise	7,921	9,783	10,579
Founded – Cleared by Charge	3,558	4,060	4,257

Of note, when considering all founded files for each year, the proportion of founded – not cleared files decreased each year from 22% in 2009 to 20% in 2010 and 19% in 2011. Correspondingly, the proportion of founded – cleared otherwise increased from 54% in 2009 to 57% in 2010 and 58% in

2011. The proportion of founded – cleared by charge remained relatively stable with a high of 24% in 2009 to a low of 23% in 2011. Moreover, the overwhelming explanation for founded —cleared otherwise files was departmental discretion. In fact, for the three years under consideration, virtually all (approximately 98%) of all founded—cleared otherwise files were coded as departmental discretion.

A further refinement of the data was done to determine how many founded files had only a marihuana possession UCR code (see Table 3). In other words, the data presented in Table 3 reflects the proportion of founded files by year in which the only offence was possession of marihuana or, as per UCR survey rules, a traffic offence was also part of the incident and two police files were made to record each offence separately. As demonstrated by Table 3, the proportions remained very stable over the three years under review. Importantly, similar to the data presented in Table 2, while the raw number of files increased slightly in each of the three years, the general ways in which these files were resolved remained extremely consistent. Critically, when marihuana possession was the only charge, these cases are very infrequently cleared by charge.

TABLE 3: *Proportion of Founded Files with Only a Marihuana Possession UCR Code*

CCJS Code	2009	2010	2011
Founded – Not Cleared	32%	29%	27%
Founded – Cleared Otherwise	65%	68%	70%
Founded – Cleared by Charge	3%	3%	3%

The total proportion of files that had a marihuana UCR code either on its own or in combination with other UCR codes, and had a CDSA charge approved by Crown, decreased over the three year period under review from 27% in 2009 to a slight increase to 28% in 2010, and finally down to its lowest proportion of 25.2% in 2011. Of note, the data extraction from PRIME did not differentiate what drug the charge was associated to. Therefore, the number of charges sworn may include possession of drugs listed in other schedules, as well as trafficking offences, production, import/export, and marihuana possession offences. Still, in terms of raw numbers of files, there were only very minor increases from 2009 to 2010, and then a minor decrease from 2010 to 2011 in the number of files associated to having an information sworn with a CDSA undetermined drug, including trafficking charge, the number of CDSA undetermined drug, including trafficking charges laid, the number of CDSA charges for drug possession (drug undetermined), and the number of CDSA charges for possession for the purposes of trafficking (drug undetermined) (see Table 4). In effect, with the exception of the number of CDSA charges for possession for the purpose of trafficking (drug undetermined), there were only slight increases in the number of files from 2009 to 2011. And, with respect to files for possession for the purposes of trafficking, the raw number of files in 2011 was at its lowest over the three years under review.

Table 4: *Charges Laid by Crown in Relation to a File with a Marihuana Possession UCR Code*

	2009	2010	2011
Files Where an Information was Sworn with a CDSA Charge	969	1,144	1,072
Total Number of CDSA Charges Laid	1,533	1,762	1,638
Number of CDSA Charges for Possession	1,123	1,311	1,261
Number of CDSA Charges for Possession for the Purpose of Trafficking	289	307	266

In terms of how the courts adjudicated these files, Table 5 presents the outcomes over the 3 years under review. It is important to keep in mind that this data represents the court outcomes for how charges proceeded through the court process for any cases where the police indicated marihuana possession as one of the UCR codes and inclusive of any other charge that may have been part of the specific police file. For example, if a person was charged with possession of cocaine and they also had a small amount of marihuana, the police file would have a UCR code for both; however, the court outcome data obtained from PRIME will only show that a CDSA charge was laid without distinguishing what drug may have been the basis for the charge. Again, the results presented in Table 5 are very consistent over the three years; however, it is interesting to note that the proportion of cases that resulted in a conviction decreased in each of the three years reviewed from a high of 28% in 2009 to a low of 19% in 2011. It is also relevant that nearly one-third of files each year were stayed, withdrawn, or dismissed.

TABLE 5: *Outcome of CDSA Charges from a File with a Marihuana Possession UCR Code*

Outcome	2009 (n = 1,533)	2010 (n = 1,762)	2011 (n = 1,638)
Guilty of Lesser Offence	1%	1%	1%
Extra-Judicial Measures/Diversion	3%	3%	2%
Not Guilty/Acquitted/Absolute Discharge	2%	2%	2%
Conditional Discharge	3%	4%	3%
Convicted	28%	25%	19%
No Charge/Crown Would Not Prosecute	18%	23%	20%
Stayed/Withdrawn/Dismissed	38%	31%	30%
Still in Progress	6%	11%	23%

In terms of the types of dispositions associated with a conviction for a marihuana possession file, over the three years under review, on average, slightly less than one-quarter (18 per cent) of convictions resulted in a prison term. In terms of the general pattern of incarceration, 2009 has 21% of convictions result in some term of imprisonment. This decreased to 16% in 2010, but slightly increased to 17% in 2011. In considering just 2011, the data suggests that of the 4,257 cleared by charge files, 305 resulted in a conviction, and, of those convicted, 53 resulted in a prison sentence. However, the data does not indicate whether the possession of marihuana or some other offence was responsible for the custody disposition.

When considering just the 2011 data for files with only a marihuana possession UCR code cleared by charge (3 per cent or 249 files), slightly more than two-thirds (68 per cent) proceeded to court. Of these, 24% or 42 files resulted in a conviction. The same proportion resulted in no charge, a smaller proportion resulted in a stay of proceedings (19 per cent), and nearly one-third (32 per cent) resulted in some other disposition. In other words, in 2011, in British Columbia, only 42 files that only had possession of marihuana as the sole charge resulted in a conviction with some kind of disposition. Critically, only seven of these 42 files resulted in any type of custody sentence. More specifically, four of these seven files resulted in a jail term of only one day, two files resulted in a jail term of seven days, and one file resulted in 14 days in jail. In summary, very few files in which possession of marihuana was the only or most serious offence was cleared by charge (3 per cent), and of those, a very small proportion resulted in a conviction of some kind (17 per cent). Of those, a very small proportion was associated with a jail term (17 per cent), and those that did result in jail had very short custody terms (X^2 = 4.6 days).

CPIC criminal records check of those who were convicted and sentenced to custody for possession of marihuana, regardless of whether there were other charges associated to the conviction, indicated that the overwhelmingly majority of offenders were male (95 per cent) and, on average, 33 years old. Moreover, these individuals were typically prolific offenders with criminal histories spanning, on average, 12 years with 19 prior convictions (see Table 6). As such, it appears that one's criminal history contributed to a custody sentence when marihuana possession was either the only charge or a concurrent charge, rather than the assumption stated in the introduction that many people are sentenced to custody exclusively because they were found to be in possession of marihuana.

TABLE 6: *Criminal Histories of Offenders Sentenced to Custody in BC for Possession of Marihuana (n = 155)*

	Per Cent or Number	Average Number of Prior Offences
Male	95%	
Average Age	33 Years Old	
Prior Criminal History	90%	19
Average Length of Criminal History	12 Years	
Convictions for Property Offences	75%	8
Convictions for Violent Offences	64%	3
Convictions for Non-Compliance	74%	4
Convictions for Criminal Driving Offences	30%	1
Convictions for Drug Offences	64%	3
Average Number of Jurisdictions Charged In	4	
Served a Previous Prison Sentence	83%	
Prolific Offender (10 or More Prior Convictions)	57%	

What garners the most attention from researchers, advocates, and policy makers are marihuana possession files that are cleared by charge. Of all the founded marihuana possession files from 2009 to 2011, nearly one-quarter (24 per cent) were categorized as founded—cleared by charge. Over the three years under review, this averaged nearly 4,000 incidents per year in which a charge of some type was forwarded to Crown Counsel or a provincial violation ticket was issued for a concurrent offence related to marihuana possession. This average is higher than the numbers provided by Statistics Canada because they only receive information from the primary UCR line in PRIME, or the offence considered the most serious. The analysis in this report examined all four UCR lines in PRIME and used any file in which marihuana possession was indicated.

For a marihuana possession file to be reported to CCJS, their reporting criteria requires that marihuana possession must be in the primary UCR field; however, this current study included all marihuana possession incidents recorded in any of the UCR fields. As demonstrated in Table 7, this results in a greater number of total files considered in each of the three years under review, and likely give a more accurate accounting of the number of marihuana possession incidents cleared by charge. The small number of files cleared by charge in which marihuana possession was the only UCR code suggests that police are rarely recommending a charge in incidents where there is no concurrent offence.

Table 7: *Comparison of Cleared by Charge Incidents by UCR Field*

	2009	2010	2011
Cleared by Charge Incident (Marihuana Possession as Primary UCR Code)	3,246	3,626	3,774
Cleared by Charge Incidents (Marihuana Possession in any UCR Field)	3,558	4,060	4,257
Marihuana Possession as the only UCR Code	183	237	249

Due to a variety of limitations with extracting specific data from PRIME, it was only determined if a CDSA charge of any type resulted from the incident. For the files reported to CCJS, this should not present a major problem, as all drug offences, except the possession of ecstasy, are considered more serious than marihuana possession by CCJS. Since the reportable incidents to CCJS have marihuana possession as the primary UCR code, it can be assumed that most of the CDSA charges are for possession of marihuana. As demonstrated by Table 8, on average, slightly more than one-quarter (27 per cent) of founded – cleared by charge incidents have an actual CDSA charge that is sworn and initiates the court process. This represents a reduction by approximately two-thirds in the number of marihuana possession charges reported by Statistics Canada.

TABLE 8: *Comparison of Cleared by Charge Files and Sworn CDSA Charges*

	2009	2010	2011
Marihuana Possession Police Files Founded—Cleared by Charge	3,558	4,060	4,257
Number of Police Files with a CDSA Charge Sworn	969	1,144	1,072
Proportion of Founded—Cleared by Charge Marihuana Possession Files that Proceed to a Sworn Charge	27%	28%	25%

The outcome of incidents that involved a CDSA charge, and possibly other charges, suggests that, on average, 388 convictions result from the average 4,000 marihuana possession files categorized as cleared by charge. Again, these 388 convictions represent convictions of any type and not necessarily for marihuana possession. These convictions were further examined to determine which incidents led to a prison sentence. On average, 18% of those convicted resulted in a prison sentence. Again, it is important to emphasize that the conviction and/or prison sentence may not be due primarily or at all to a marihuana possession offence. Accordingly, in 2011, of the 14,836 marihuana possession incidents that had evidence against a known person, a total of 305 incidents resulted in a conviction for a drug offence that was not necessarily a marihuana possession offence. Of those convicted, in 2011, 53 resulted in a prison sentence.

Recommendations and Conclusion

The data published by Statistics Canada regarding the number of people charged for marihuana possession offences in British Columbia is a gross over count of people actually being charged. According to Statistics Canada, the definition of cleared by charge states that at least one accused must have been identified and either a charge was laid or recommended against an individual in connection with the incident. These criteria complicate police file scoring as it relates to marihuana possession data because the rule does not specify that the charge laid has to be for the offence listed in the primary UCR field. In cases where a less serious criminal or CDSA offence is listed in one of the non-primary UCR fields, the cleared by charge status may refer to that offence. Furthermore, the charge may also be a provincial statute charge, such as a violation ticket for being intoxicated in public. It is easy to conceive of instances where a police officer processes a person for a liquor act violation who is also in possession of marihuana may give a warning for the drug offence and issue a violation ticket for the provincial offence. The file status would indicate 'charged' in reference to the violation ticket; however, PRIME would automatically place the marihuana offence as the primary offence.

The 4,257 incidents from PRIME and the 3,774 incidents reported by Statistics Canada in 2011 that are listed as cleared by charge do not accurately represent that number of marihuana possession incidents that are actually proceeding by charge. In fact, only 1,072 incidents proceeded with a drug charge being sworn and this is not necessarily for marihuana possession. This indicates that all of the other incidents were being charged in some other manner, most likely through a provincial offence. The inaccurate cleared by charge classification given to the majority of marihuana possession incidents is alarming, and has greater implications when considering the prospect of this occurring with other criminal offences; for example, an assault incident that does not proceed to charge is classified as cleared by charge due to a liquor act ticket being issued to address the concurrent offence within the incident.

The fact that approximately 70% of marihuana possession incidents that are cleared by charge or otherwise are done so by departmental discretion implies that police are, in most cases, concluding the marihuana offence with a verbal warning. It is suggested that this is an under estimation of the police discretion to not proceed by charge, as supported by the small amount of formal charges laid on all incidents involving marihuana possession. In 2011, of the 14,836 opportunities for police in British Columbia to charge a person for marihuana possession, only 7% of incidents resulted in a criminal charge of some kind and only 2% resulted in a conviction. The low rate of charges associated to marihuana possession offences clearly indicates that the possession of marihuana results in little formal consequences beyond the loss of the marihuana. This may be a factor in the increased public tolerance for the drug. The lack of response to marihuana possession may serve as a message from the government that they find it acceptable for people to possess marihuana, but are reluctant to make formal changes to legalize the substance.

In conclusion, less than 1% of all marihuana possession seizures in British Columbia in 2011 resulted in someone receiving a prison sentence, and not necessarily for the possession of marihuana. In fact, in 2011, only 249 files had possession of marihuana was the only or most serious offence and, in these cases, only seven files resulted in a jail term, which was typically either one day or seven days in length. Police are rarely recommending charges when they encounter people with marihuana. Moreover, when charges are recommended, there are usually other offences being committed in addition to the possession of marihuana and the individuals have long criminal histories, which contribute to the decision to recommend charges. Contrary to an acceptance of the data as presented by Statistics Canada, thoughtful consideration of the limitations and challenges associated with this data and a more nuanced examination of the files indicates that, at least in British Columbia, there are not thousands of people being charged and convicted of possession of marihuana. Instead, the vast majority of these cases, when founded, are not cleared by charge, and for the small proportion that are cleared by charge, very rarely do these files result in a conviction and jail time. Before policy-makers and the public decide on the most appropriate ways to respond to all of the complicated issues involved with marihuana, an important first step is to understand the reality of marihuana possession in British Columbia.

References

Auditor General of Canada. (2001). *Report of the Auditor General: Exhibit 11.2—Number of Persons Charged for Offences Under the Controlled Drugs and Substances Act in Canada during 1999*. Retrieved from: http://www.oag-bvg.gc.ca/internet/English/att_0111xe02_e_11630.html.

Boyd, N. (2013). *The Enforcement of Marijuana Possession Offences in British Columbia: A Blueprint for Change*. Simon Fraser University.

Canadian Centre for Justice Statistics. (2013). *Uniform Crime Reporting Incident-Based Survey*. Updated January 7, 2013.

Hollins, D. (2007). *Strategies for Clearance Rate Improvements in "E" Division RCMP*. Prepared by the Operations Strategy Branch, "E" Division RCMP.

Liberal Party of Canada. (2013). *Legalization of Marijuana: Answering Questions and Developing a Framework – Draft January 2013*. Retrieved from: https://bc.liberal.ca/files/2013/01/DRAFT-Marijuana-Policy-Paper-Jan-13.pdf

Mahony, T.H. and Turner, J. (2010). Police-Reported Clearance Rates in Canada, 2010. Statistics Canada. Retrieved from: http://www.statcan.gc.ca/pub/85-002-x/2012001/article/11647-eng.htm

McCormick, A.V., Haarhoff, T., Cohen, I.M., Plecas, D., & Burk, K. (2010). *Challenges Associated with Interpreting and Using Police Clearance Rates*. University of the Fraser Valley.

Ministry of Justice, Police Service Division. (2012). *Crime Statistics and British Columbia, 2011*. Retrieved from: http://www.pssg.gov.bc.ca/policeservices/shareddocs/crime-statistics.pdf

Special Committee on Illegal Drugs (2002) *Final Report: Our Position for a Canadian Public Policy*. Retrieved from: http://www.parl.gc.ca/SenCommitteeBusiness/CommitteeReports.aspx?parl=37&ses=1&comm_id=85

Statistics Canada. (2011). *Police-Reported Crime for Selected Offences, Canada, 2010 and 2011*. Retrieved from: http://www.statcan.gc.ca/pub/85-002-x/2012001/article/11692/tbl/tbl04-eng.htm

Vancouver Sun. (2012). *Pot Possession Charges in B.C. Up 88% Over Last Decade.* Published November 4, 2012. Retrieved from: http://www.vancouversun.com/news/possession+charges+cent+years/7492120/story.html

Kale Pauls has been a member of the RCMP for 10 years and has provided expert opinions for the courts on marihuana and other drug trafficking offences. He has worked in general duty, drug enforcement, mental-health crisis response, and serious crime sections. Kale hold a BA from Simon Fraser University and a MA in Criminal Justice from the University of the Fraser Valley.

Dr. Darryl Plecas is Professor Emeritus at the School of Criminology and Criminal Justice, University of the Fraser Valley. He is the author or co-author of more than 200 research reports and publications addressing a broad range of criminal justice issues. He holds two degrees in criminology from Simon Fraser University, and a doctorate in Higher Education from the University of British Columbia. He is currently the Member of the Legislative Assembly for British Columbia representing Abbotsford South and Parliamentary Secretary for Crime Reduction to the Minister of Justice.

Dr. Irwin M. Cohen is a faculty member in the School of Criminology and Criminal Justice at the University of the Fraser Valley, the holder of the University Senior Research Chair, RCMP for Crime Reduction, and the Director of the Centre for Public Safety and Criminal Justice Research. He received his PhD from Simon Fraser University. Dr. Cohen has also published many scholarly articles and book chapters, delivered many lectures, conference papers, and workshops, and written policy reports on a wide range of topics including policing issues, restorative justice, serious and violent young offenders, Aboriginal victimization issues, and terrorism.

Tara Haarhoff is currently the Senior Data Analyst with the Criminal Analysis Section of the 'E' Division Royal Canadian Mounted Police (RCMP). She also holds the position of RCMP Liaison for the University Led Research Program. Since 2003, she has served as a Research Associate with the Centre for Public Safety and Criminal Justice Research in the School of Criminology and Criminal Justice at the University of the Fraser Valley. She is a member of the British Columbia Crime Statistics Committee and the International Association of Crime Analysts. She has authored and co-authored numerous research reports on a broad range of policing issues. Tara graduated with a Master of Arts Degree in Criminal Justice from the University of the Fraser Valley in June of 2011 and is currently enrolled in the Crime & Intelligence Analysis Advanced Specialty Certificate Program at the British Columbia Institute of Technology.